Frailty and Sarcopenia - Recent Evidence and New Perspectives

Edited by Grazia D'Onofrio and Julianna Cseri

Published in London, United Kingdom

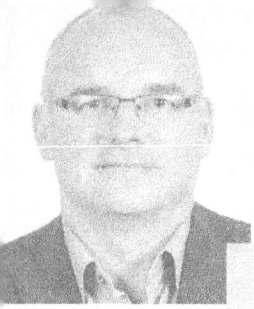
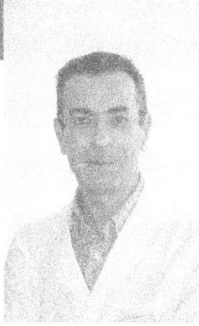
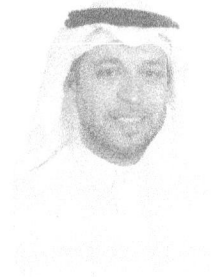
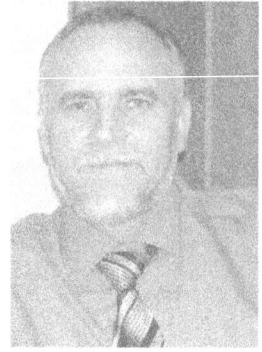
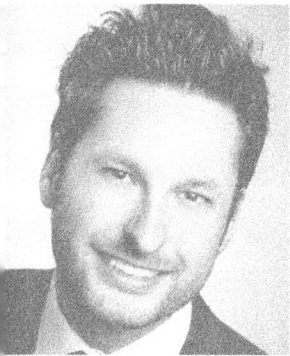
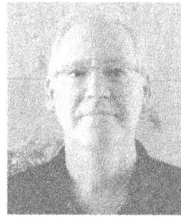
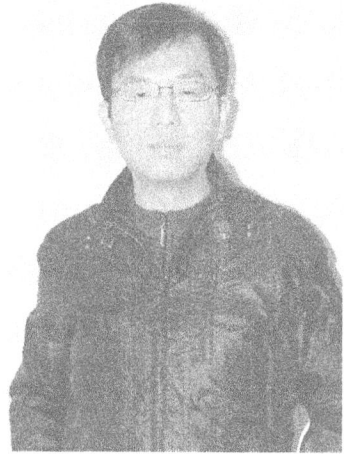

IntechOpen

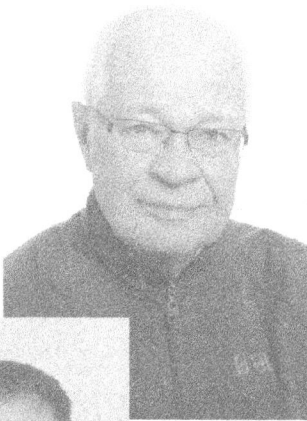
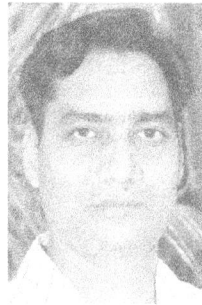
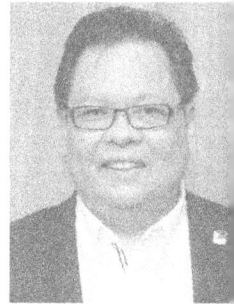
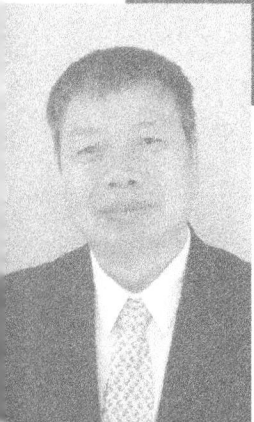
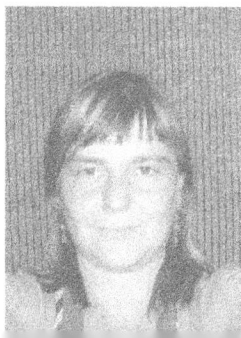
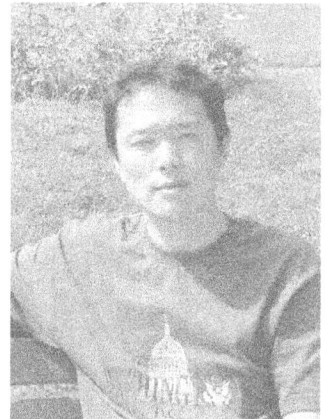

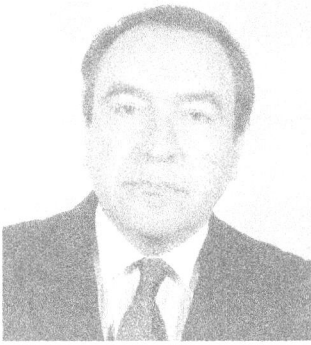

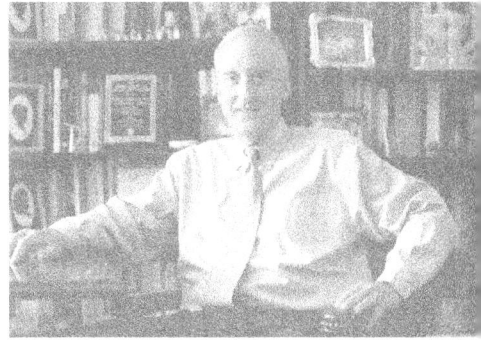

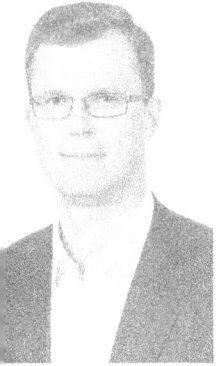

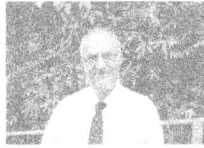

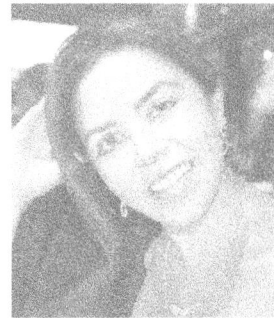

Supporting open minds since 2005

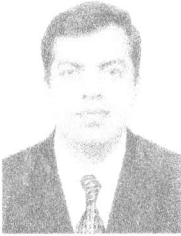

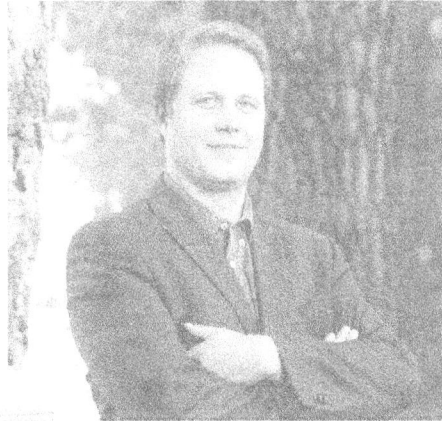

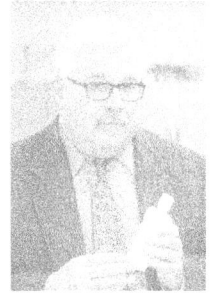

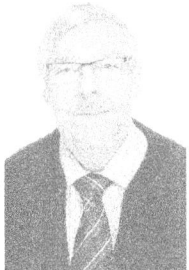

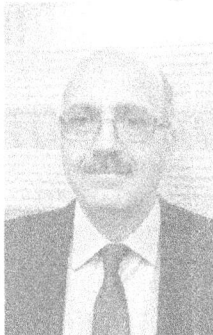

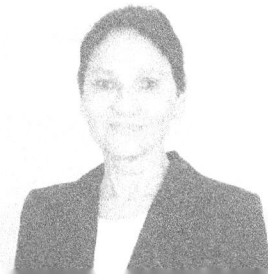

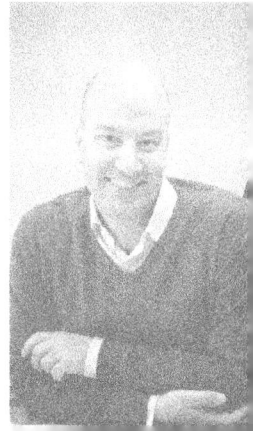

Frailty and Sarcopenia - Recent Evidence and New Perspectives
http://dx.doi.org/10.5772/intechopen.95708
Edited by Grazia D'Onofrio and Julianna Cseri

Contributors
Charles Lambert, Norihide Fukushima, Jia-Ping Wu, Tiago Fernandes, Bruno Rocha de Avila Pelozin, Luis Felipe Rodrigues, Edilamar Menezes De Oliveira, Carlos Sáez, Sara García-Isidoro, Grazia D'Onofrio

Notice
Statements and opinions expressed in the chapters are these of the individual contributors and not necessarily those of the editors or publisher. No responsibility is accepted for the accuracy of information contained in the published chapters. The publisher assumes no responsibility for any damage or injury to persons or property arising out of the use of any materials, instructions, methods or ideas contained in the book.

First published in London, United Kingdom, 2022 by IntechOpen
IntechOpen is the global imprint of INTECHOPEN LIMITED, registered in England and Wales, registration number: 11086078, 5 Princes Gate Court, London, SW7 2QJ, United Kingdom
Printed in Croatia

British Library Cataloguing-in-Publication Data
A catalogue record for this book is available from the British Library

Additional hard and PDF copies can be obtained from orders@intechopen.com

Frailty and Sarcopenia - Recent Evidence and New Perspectives
Edited by Grazia D'Onofrio and Julianna Cseri
p. cm.
Print ISBN 978-1-80355-021-3
Online ISBN 978-1-80355-022-0
eBook (PDF) ISBN 978-1-80355-023-7

We are IntechOpen,
the world's leading publisher of
Open Access books
Built by scientists, for scientists

6,000+
Open access books available

148,000+
International authors and editors

185M+
Downloads

Our authors are among the

156
Countries delivered to

Top 1%
most cited scientists

12.2%
Contributors from top 500 universities

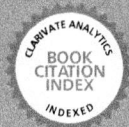

Interested in publishing with us?
Contact book.department@intechopen.com

Numbers displayed above are based on latest data collected.
For more information visit www.intechopen.com

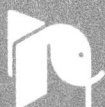

Meet the editors

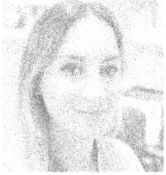

Dr. Grazia D'Onofrio is a psychologist and researcher in the Health Department, Scientific Institute for Research and Clinical Care (IRCCS) "Casa Sollievo della Sofferenza," Italy. In 2009 she was awarded the title of Expert in Integrated Psychodynamic Psychotherapy. In 2020 she obtained a Ph.D. in Biorobotics. She is the author of several scientific articles, reviews, book chapters, and abstracts presented at medical congresses. Currently, she is an editorial board member for some international journals and a guest editor for special issues about Alzheimer's disease. Her research interests include aging, dementia, psychological and behavioural symptoms, multidimensional impairment, information and communication technologies, and Ambient Assisted Living.

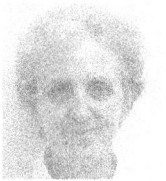

Julianna Cseri, MD, Ph.D., was a college professor who retired from the Department of Physiotherapy, Faculty of Public Health, University of Debrecen, Hungary. Her scientific field was skeletal muscle physiology. She was awarded her general medicine diploma in 1973 from the University Medical School of Debrecen and started scientific work at the Department of Physiology, University Medical School of Debrecen (later the Faculty of Medicine University of Debrecen). She achieved scientific qualification in muscle electrophysiology. Her attention was later turned to the proliferation and differentiation of the skeletal muscle in cell cultures and the role of intracellular calcium homeostasis in myogenesis. This work is closely related to muscle degeneration and regeneration in vivo, managed by physiotherapy interventions.

Contents

Preface

Interest in the frail elderly, or rather the concept of frailty, is increasing as the aging population continues to grow. The Latin writer Publio Terenzio Afro stated in the comedy *Formione*, "*Senectus ipsa est morbus*" ("old age is a disease in itself"). Of the opposite opinion is Cicero, who in *De senectute* exalts the advantages of the third age. Undoubtedly, frailty is a dynamic condition of increased vulnerability, reflecting age-related pathophysiological changes of a multisystemic nature, associated with an increased risk of adverse outcomes, such as institutionalization, hospitalization, and death. Having ascertained that frailty in the elderly is determined by a disorder of multiple physiological systems that interact with each other, we can make two basic assumptions:

1. Frailty is a physiological syndrome characterized by the reduction of functional reserves and the decreased resistance to stressors resulting from the cumulative decline of multiple physiological systems.

2. Frailty is a dynamic state that affects an individual who experiences losses in one or more functional domains (physical, psychic, social).

Regardless of the operational definitions, in the frail elderly, the physiological reduction of the body's homeostatic mechanisms occurs in an accelerated and clinically detectable manner as pathological. Aging is accompanied by a progressive decrease in muscle mass known as sarcopenia, which limits autonomy and makes elderly people more vulnerable to external aggressions. Sarcopenia can affect 20% of the population between the ages of 65 and 70 and up to 40% of over-octogenarians and can be associated with alterations in the individual's immunological capacity. The effects of poor nutrition and sarcopenia overlap, contributing to the functional decline of the musculoskeletal system, responsible for impaired gait and balance correlated with a high risk of falls and fractures.

The disease thus becomes an integral part of everyday life and the elderly feel even weaker, less efficient, and of great burden to the family.

The highly negative impact of multidimensional risk compromised of isolation and mortality confirms that fragility is the most common condition associated with mortality in the elderly. Low levels of activity and decreased protein and micronutrient intake in the diet can unleash fragility and accelerate it. For these reasons, it becomes crucial in clinical practice to identify, measure, and treat frailty. The primary objective of treatment is the preservation of maximum personal and social autonomy. Proper nutrition characterized by a sufficient energy intake and associated with the implementation of protein intake and targeted and constant physical exercise can promote the health and autonomy of the elderly and prevent serious complications.

This book is an up-to-date and realistic view on physiopathological mechanisms, assessment tools, and rehabilitation activities of sarcopenia in frail elderly. It includes topical contributions from multiple disciplines to support the fundamental goals of extending active life and enhancing its quality.

Grazia D'Onofrio
Clinical Psychology Service,
Health Department,
Fondazione IRCCS Casa Sollievo Della Sofferenza,
San Giovanni Rotondo, Italy

Note from the Publisher

It is with great sadness and regret that we inform the future readers of this book that the editor, Prof. Julianna Cseri, passed away shortly before finishing the book and having a chance to see its publication.

Prof. Julianna Cseri was IntechOpen's dear collaborator and she authored 1 book chapter with us and edited 2 books, "Background and Management of Muscular Atrophy" and "Skeletal Muscle - From Myogenesis to Clinical Relations".

This collaboration continued until her final days when she was acting as the editor of the book "Frailty and Sarcopenia - Recent Evidence and New Perspectives".

We would like to acknowledge Prof. Julianna Cseri contribution to open access scientific publishing, which she made during the years of dedicated work, and express our gratitude for her pleasant cooperation with us.

IntechOpen Team, September 2022

Section 1

Introduction

Introductory Chapter: Frailty and Sarcopenia – Recent Evidence and New Perspectives

Grazia D'Onofrio

1. Introduction

Frailty refers to a state of increased vulnerability and reduced resilience to stressful events. Sarcopenia, on the other hand, is a syndrome characterized by progressive and generalized loss of musculoskeletal mass and function (muscle strength or physical performance), with an increased risk of adverse outcomes (falls, fractures, hospitalization, worse quality of life, and mortality). These two conditions actually present large overlaps. The sarcopenia, in fact, constitutes an essential component within the physical model of frailty proposed by Fried (involuntary weight loss, muscle weakness, slowed walking speed, reduced physical activity, exhaustion) [1]. This physical phenotype can be in turn inserted, as suggested by Rockwood, in a larger multidimensional model of frailty, comprising psychological and social aspects, multi-morbidity, and disability [2, 3].

Currently, sarcopenia is considered a true and own biological substrate of physical frailty. Loss of muscle mass typically begins in the fifth decade of life and proceeds with a falling speed of 0.8% per year [4]. Epidemiological data suggest wide prevalence variability, depending on population type study, gender, age, setting, and diagnostic criteria used. According to a recent review, comprising 5 European clinical trials, the prevalence of sarcopenia is 7.5% (elderly subjects in community) to 77.6% (patients in rehabilitation/convalescence) [5].

Sarcopenia can occur in sedentary subjects as a result of a long period of physical inactivity [6] or it can be accentuated simply by the onset of old age [7–9]. According to current studies, sarcopenia is not an inevitable consequence of age but occurs under conditions of oxidative stress, increasing over time with the formation of free radicals.

Regarding sarcopenia linked to the third age in the male sex, is related to the decrease in the production of testosterone that has anabolic effects, in particular on protein metabolism.

In sarcopenia, the loss of muscle mass and the consequent loss of strength are also accompanied by reduced muscle function. In general, sarcopenia produces a deterioration of physical functions and also means:

- Postural instability.

- Changes in thermoregulation (increased mortality in extreme summer or winter).

- Worse bone trophism (lack of stimulation of contraction).

• Modification of glucidic homeostasis (lack of storage and consumption).

• Reduction in basal energy production.

With the passing of the years of life of a standard subject (considered as an examination sample) the loss of muscle mass advances in step with the loss of muscle strength that can be of the same or even greater proportions. At 50 years of age, many people have already lost about 10% of their muscle mass and at 70 years of age, they will have lost about 70% [10].

The effects of sarcopenia contribute to the functional decline of the musculo-skeletal system, responsible for impaired gait and balance and a high risk of falls and consequent serious fractures [11]. The disease thus becomes an integral part of everyday life and the elderly feel even weaker, less efficient, and of great weight for the family.

The highly negative impact of multidimensional compromise on the risk of isolation and mortality confirms that frailty is the most common condition associated with mortality in the elderly. Low levels of activity and decreased protein and micronutrient intake in the diet can trigger and accelerate it. For these reasons in clinical practice, it becomes crucial to identify, measure and treat frailty.

Primary objective of care is the preservation of maximum autonomy personal and social. Proper nutrition characterized by a sufficient energy intake and associated with the implementation of protein intake and targeted and constant exercise can encourage the health conditions and autonomy of the subject elderly and prevent serious complications.

2. Classification and pathophysiology of sarcopenia

Sarcopenia is a frequent condition in the elderly but can also be observed in younger individuals. Sarcopenia can be considered "primitive" (or age-related) when no cause is highlighted if not aging, while it is considered "Secondary" when one or more causes are identifiable [8].

Muscle trophism is a consequence of a balance between anabolic stimuli (insulin, exercise, amino acids, testosterone, adrenaline, growth hormone) and catabolic stimuli (cortisol, catecholamines, glucagon, cytokines, intense exercise) [12]. It has been seen in the elderly how it tends to be there, associated with the normal aging process, a prevalence of the catabolic state which becomes predominant if there are particular conditions such as comorbidity [12]. In these cases also muscle mass suffers effects of the general catabolic state in which the organism is found [12].

From a pathophysiological point of view, they are several factors that can contribute to the development of sarcopenia [13]. Among the main ones recognized causes include:

• reduction of the growth hormone levels and insuline-like growth factor (IGF-1)

• Reduced levels of sex hormones

• Neuromuscular changes

• Physical inactivity

• Malnutrition

- Increased production of cytokines, such as Interleukin-1 (IL-1), Interleukin-6 (IL-6), tumor necrosis factor-α (TNF-α), etc.

- Alteration of the cellular redox state.

Medicines can also play a role in a protective or causative sense in the development of sarcopenia. Recently Campins et al. have highlighted such as statins, sulfonylureas and glinides have potential detrimental effects on muscle metabolism while Angiotensin-converting enzyme (ACE) inhibitors, incretins, allopurinol, formoterol, and vitamin D can play a protective role on muscle function [14].

Muscle is made up of several types of fibers muscle, such as slow fibers (type I) and fast fibers (type IIa and IIb). With aging and in particular, in sarcopenic patients, there is a reduction in the diameter of the muscle fibers as well as a progressive loss of rapid fibers which translates, clinically, in a reduction of the strength, the coordination of movements, and speed of the way. This happens because the fibers lost in rapid muscles are replaced by slow fibers by motor neurons adjacent [15]. However, given the dynamic nature of the neuromuscular remodeling, it has been seen as well as the muscle of the elderly subject, under certain stimuli, maintains the ability to respond and adapt to the new state required [16]. So much so that it is proved as even just the lifestyle can greatly affect the development muscle mass [17].

It is precisely from the reversibility of the processes that lead to sarcopenia which derives the possibility of a therapeutic intervention (and still more preventive) is effective.

3. Sarcopenia and frailty

Sarcopenia is considered a key component of frailty since, by acting on the reduction of mass and power muscle, causes a reduced physical performance with a consequent reduction in walking speed up to hypo-immobility [18].

Frailty is the most problematic expression of characterized aging from a state of vulnerability to any stressful event. It is due to the reduced homeostatic reserve of the body which follows the functional decline of different physiological systems over the course of life.

These changes mean that the fragile person is exposed to disproportionate responses to the triggering event leading to important repercussions on the plan socio-sanitary.

In fact, it is demonstrated how frailty is associated with an increased risk of negative outcomes such as falls, delirium, disability, institutionalization, hospitalization, and death [19].

4. Prevention and treatment

Given the multifactorial pathogenesis of sarcopenia and the lack of knowledge of the interactions between the various causal factors, a global and standardized approach to the prevention and treatment of this condition does not exist.

It is now universally accepted and recognized that following a diet balanced and complete (Mediterranean diet) and practicing regular physical activity have a fundamental role in the prevention of sarcopenia [20]. In particular, in the elderly, scientific evidence suggests that the protein requirement in the diet has increased compared to the 0.8 g/kg required for adults [21]. On the other hand, it is very frequent to note a progressive reduction in protein intake with increasing age [22]. These cases can be considered protein integration through the administration of whole proteins or amino acids essential. Several studies have shown how important not only the quantity administered but also the modality of administration and subdivision in the day. Amino acids have a greater ability to stimulate the synthesis of protein after taking orally or intravenously compared to integration in the whole protein diet. They are also directly usable by the body without the need for additional metabolic steps. However, their effects depend on the moment of administration: if administered before physical activity they are used mainly as energy substrates while if taken after exercise they mainly contribute to the repair muscular [23]. There are several on the market both oral formulations, such as tablets, sachets, or jellies for dysphagia patients than for intravenous use. The systemic effect of administering essential amino acids has been shown to be much more ample being able because it affects metabolism glycidic and insulin resistance [24]. Also supplementation with vitamin D is considered important. More controversial is resorting to hormonal therapies, for example with estrogen and Dehydroepiandrosterone (DHEA) [25].

Exercise plays a key role in the prevention and treatment of sarcopenia and, a today, it turns out to be the most effective approach. Through the stimulus given by physical activity, numerous are activated at the muscular level pathways that converge towards anabolic pathways with positive consequences on trophism and on muscle quality. In particular, moderate resistance exercises intensity produces the greatest results in elderly and/or sarcopenic subjects [26]. Particularly intense exercise is not beneficial further benefits if not actually harmful.

Due to the multifaceted nature of sarcopenia, the best therapeutic approach can only be multidisciplinary, requiring collaboration between different figures specialists such as the geriatrician, the internist, the physiatrist, the general practitioner, the nutritionist, and physiotherapist.

In addition, the nutritional aspect is important and not only intended as a protein supplement. In fact, elderly patients often have unbalanced diet, and a nutritional assessment with the advice of a specific diet is essential [21, 27]. Once you have all the information from anamnestic and necessary clinics comes a personalized rehabilitation plan is recommended, which also takes into account any clinical conditions that may limit or contraindicate certain exercises. Like this, depending on the individual patient, they come recommended exercises to be performed in the gym either at home or cycles are prescribed rehabilitation to be performed on an outpatient basis through a specific machine. The follow-up includes a control outpatient periodical with a re-evaluation of physical performance to monitor the progress and make any changes to rehabilitation plans.

5. Conclusion

Sarcopenia is a morbid condition that involves the skeletal musculature and has repercussions on a multisystem level. It is a chronic but reversible process as well as preventable. The most effective approach consists in exercising appropriately supplemented by nutritional supplementation, in particular with essential amino acids. The hope is that efforts will be intensified in prevention, through lifestyle changes, and in the implementation of screening for an early diagnosis of sarcopenia, a very pathological condition underestimated as widespread.

Author details

Grazia D'Onofrio
Clinical Psychology Service, Health Department, Fondazione IRCCS Casa Sollievo della Sofferenza, Foggia, Italy

*Address all correspondence to: graziadonofrio@libero.it

IntechOpen

References

[1] Fried LP. Conference on the physiologic basis of frailty. April 28, 1992, Baltimore, Maryland, U.S.A. Introduction. Aging (Milano). 1992;**4**(3):251-252

[2] Rockwood K, Fox RA, Stolee P, Robertson D, Beattie BL. Frailty in elderly people: An evolving concept. CMAJ. 1994;**150**(4):489-495

[3] Cruz-Jentoft AJ, Kiesswetter E, Drey M, Sieber CC. Nutrition, frailty, and sarcopenia. Aging Clinical and Experimental Research. 2017;**29**(1): 43-48

[4] Landi F, Calvani R, Cesari M, Tosato M, Martone AM, Bernabei R, et al. Sarcopenia as the Biological Substrate of Physical Frailty. Clinics in Geriatric Medicine. 2015;**31**(3):367-374

[5] Lardiés Sánchez B, Sanz-París A, Boj-Carceller D, Cruz-Jentoft AJ. Systematic review: Prevalence of sarcopenia in ageing people using bioelectrical impedance analysis to assess muscle mass. European Geriatric Medicine. 2016;7:256-261

[6] Derbré F, Gratas-Delamarche A, Gómez-Cabrera MC, Viña J. Inactivity-induced oxidative stress: A central role in age-related sarcopenia? European Journal of Sport Science. 2014;**14** (Suppl. 1):S98-S108

[7] Morley JE, Kim MJ, Haren MT, Kevorkian R, Banks WA. Frailty and the aging male. The Aging Male. 2005;**8**:135-140

[8] Cruz-Jentoft AJ, Baeyens JP, Bauer JM, Boirie Y, Cederholm T, Landi F, et al. European working group on sarcopenia in older people. Sarcopenia: European consensus on definition and diagnosis: Report of the European working group on sarcopenia in older people. Age and Ageing. 2010;**39**:412-423

[9] Muscaritoli M, Anker SD, Argilés J, Aversa Z, Bauer JM, Biolo G, et al. Consensus definition of sarcopenia, cachexia and pre-cachexia: Joint document elaborated by Special Interest Groups (SIG) "cachexia-anorexia in chronic wasting diseases" and "nutrition in geriatrics". Clinical Nutrition. 2010;**29**:154-159

[10] Padilla Colón CJ, Molina-Vicenty IL, Frontera-Rodríguez M, García-Ferré A, Rivera BP, Cintrón-Vélez G, et al. Muscle and bone mass loss in the elderly population: Advances in diagnosis and treatment. Journal of Biomedicine. 2018;**3**:40-49

[11] Narici MV, Maffulli N. Sarcopenia: Characteristics, mechanisms and functional significance. British Medical Bulletin. 2010;**95**:139-159

[12] McCarthy JJ, Esser KA. Anabolic and catabolic pathways regulating skeletal muscle mass. Current Opinion in Clinical Nutrition and Metabolic Care. 2010;**13**(3):230-235

[13] Lim JY, Frontera WR. Single skeletal muscle fiber mechanical properties: A muscle quality biomarker of human aging. European Journal of Applied Physiology. 2022;**122**(6):1383-1395

[14] Campins L, Camps M, Riera A, Pleguezuelos E, Yebenes JC, Serra-Prat M. Oral drugs related with muscle wasting and sarcopenia. A review. Pharmacology. 2017;**99**:1-8

[15] Kung TA, Cederna PS, van der Meulen JH, Urbanchek MG, Kuzon WM Jr, Faulkner JA. Motor unit changes seen with skeletal muscle sarcopenia in oldest old rats. The Journals of Gerontology. Series A, Biological Sciences and Medical Sciences. 2014;**69**:657-665

[16] Osoba MY, Rao AK, Agrawal SK, Lalwani AK. Balance and gait in the elderly: A contemporary review.

Laryngoscope Investig Otolaryngol. 2019;**4**(1):143-153

[17] Bartels EM, Robertson S, Danneskiold-Samsøe B, Appleyard M, Stockmarr A. Effects of lifestyle on muscle strength in a healthy danish population. Journal of Lifestyle Medicine. 2018;**8**(1):16-22

[18] Singh M, Alexander K, Roger VL, Rihal CS, Whitson HE, Lerman A, et al. Frailty and its potential relevance to cardiovascular care. Mayo Clinic Proceedings. 2008;**83**:114-153

[19] Chen CL, Chen CM, Wang CY, Ko PW, Chen CH, Hsieh CP, et al. Frailty is associated with an increased risk of major adverse outcomes in elderly patients following surgical treatment of hip fracture. Scientific Reports. 2019;**9**(1):19135

[20] Ganapathy A, Nieves JW. Nutrition and sarcopenia—What do we know? Nutrients. 2020;**12**(6):1755

[21] Baum JI, Kim IY, Wolfe RR. Protein consumption and the elderly: What is the optimal level of intake? Nutrients. 2016;**8**(6):359

[22] Rogeri PS, Zanella R, Martins GL, MDA G, Leite G, Lugaresi R, et al. Strategies to prevent sarcopenia in the aging process: Role of protein intake and exercise. Nutrients. 2022;**14**(1):52

[23] Hargreaves M, Spriet LL. Skeletal muscle energy metabolism during exercise. Nature Metabolism. 2020;**2**:817-828

[24] Bloomgarden Z. Diabetes and branched-chain amino acids: What is the link? Journal of Diabetes. 2018;**10**(5):350-352

[25] Huang LT, Wang JH. The therapeutic intervention of sex steroid hormones for sarcopenia. Front Med (Lausanne). 2021;**8**:739251

[26] Peterson MD, Rhea MR, Sen A, Gordon PM. Resistance exercise for muscular strength in older adults: A meta-analysis. Ageing Research Reviews. 2010;**9**(3):226-237

[27] Ahmed T, Haboubi N. Assessment and management of nutrition in older people and its importance to health. Clinical Interventions in Aging. 2010;**5**:207-216

Section 2

Epidemiology
and Assessment

Prevalence of Sarcopenia According to the Method Used to Determine Physical Performance

Carlos Sáez and Sara García-Isidoro

Abstract

Sarcopenia is currently defined as a progressive and generalized skeletal muscle disorder that occurs with advancing age and is associated with an increased likelihood of adverse outcomes. Low levels of measures for muscle strength, muscle quantity, and physical performance define sarcopenia. In this chapter, we will see that the prevalence of a low value of physical performance will be different according to the method used to measure this parameter, and thus, it would be foreseeable to think that the prevalence of sarcopenia will also be different according to the method used. However, despite the differences found in physical performance, we will show that the prevalence of sarcopenia appears to be regardless of the method used for physical performance, and therefore, how is it possible that having a significant difference in the prevalence of physical performance depending on the method chosen, the prevalence of sarcopenia has an almost perfect agreement? To answer these questions, a new simplified model is studied, defining sarcopenia as low muscle strength and low muscle mass and without taking physical performance into account. Finally, we will see that, indeed, physical performance does not seem to be decisive or necessary for the diagnosis of sarcopenia.

Keywords: aging, prevalence, diagnosis, sarcopenia, EWGSOP

1. Introduction

1.1 Definition of sarcopenia

The term sarcopenia comes from the Greek words *"sarco,"* which means muscle, and *"penia,"* which means loss, and was used for the first time by Dr. Irwin Rosenberg, director of the "Research Center on Aging" at Boston University (USA) which in 1989 stated: *"the most dramatic and significant age-related physical decline was the loss of lean body mass"* (**Figure 1**) [1, 2].

Thus, sarcopenia was initially defined as *"normal and involuntary loss of muscle mass due to aging"* (Rosenberg, 1989).

This definition was based on the conceptual framework that states that the decline in muscle strength due to aging was due to a parallel decline in muscle mass. However, as the field of sarcopenia progressed, studies showed that the loss of age-related muscle strength outweighed the loss of muscle mass [3], so a definition of sarcopenia based only on muscle mass was not sufficient [4]. It was

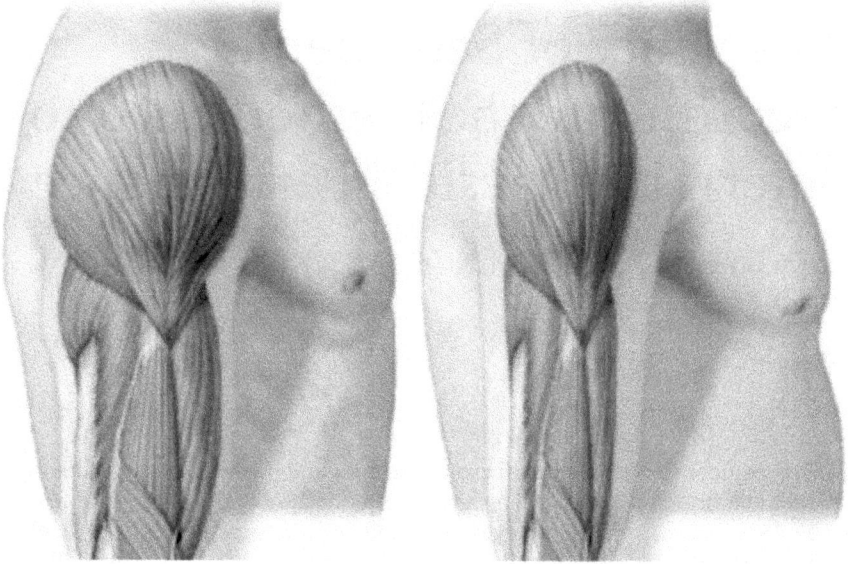

Figure 1.
Loss of muscle mass and strength due to aging (modified from: ADAM©, atlas of human anatomy. Todd R. Olson, 1997).

more precisely defined as [5]: *"Decrease in muscle mass and strength due to aging"* (Morley et al., 2001).

Since then, the number of scientific publications has increased. In those, among other findings, its possible causes and consequences were identified, and the concept of sarcopenia has evolved as different definitions emerged among researchers [6, 7]. Still, there was still a lack of a definition of sarcopenia that would be suitable both for use in research settings and in clinical practice, until significant progress was made in 2010 thanks to a joint publication by the European Working Group on Sarcopenia in Older People [8] (EWGSOP) in which sarcopenia was defined as: *"A syndrome characterized by a gradual and generalized loss of skeletal muscle mass and muscle strength with the risk of causing adverse outcomes such as physical disability, poor quality of life and even mortality"* (Cruz-Jentoft et al., 2010).

This new definition incorporated sarcopenia not only the loss of muscle mass and strength but also its consequences on physical performance [5, 9] and for many years, it was the definition that was used in most studies as a reference or *"gold standard"* for the diagnosis of sarcopenia [10].

In October 2016, the World Health Organization gave a new advance to this condition, since through the International Classification of Diseases in its 10th revision (ICD-10-CM) recognized sarcopenia not as a geriatric syndrome but as a disease (muscular), with the code M62.84 [11, 12]. This forced it to revise and update its definition again.

In the 10 years passed since the initial work of the European group in 2010, researchers and clinicians have explored many aspects of sarcopenia, and expert groups around the world have published complementary definitions of sarcopenia [13–15]. However, the more recent definition and the current one are the one proposed by this same group [16–21] who, in a review carried out in 2019, defined sarcopenia as *"A progressive and generalized skeletal muscle disorder that* occurs with aging and is associated with a greater probability of adverse outcomes such as falls, fractures, physical disability and even mortality" (Cruz-Jentoft et al., 2019).

Despite all these advances, international expert groups from around the world still do not reach a consensus on a definition of sarcopenia that is widely accepted, although they have agreed on the mechanisms and clinical implications of sarcopenia [22, 23] and especially in the fact that muscle mass, muscle strength, and physical performance are important components for the diagnosis of this disease and that therefore, all these parameters must be measured [4].

1.2 Clinical consequences of sarcopenia

The clinical consequences of sarcopenia are basically due to loss of strength and muscle mass, not only in terms of functional disabilities, fractures, hospitalizations, and increased mortality [24], but also in quality of life [25].

In terms of human health, sarcopenia increases the risk of falls and fractures [26, 27] and impairs the ability to carry out activities of daily living [28]; it is associated with heart disease [29], respiratory disease [15], and cognitive impairment [30]; and leads to mobility disorders [13]; it contributes to a decrease in the quality of life [31] and ultimately death [26].

1.3 Sarcopenia categories

Sarcopenia is a disease with many causes and variable outcomes. In some people, a clear and unique cause of sarcopenia can be identified, largely attributable to aging, but in other cases, other causes can be identified. In this way, defining the sarcopenia categories as primary and secondary can be useful in clinical practice [8, 16].

Sarcopenia can be considered "primary" (or age-related) when there is no obvious cause other than aging. Sarcopenia is considered "secondary" when there are one or more obvious causes other than aging [16].

Sarcopenia staging is a concept that can help to guide its clinical treatment, in this way it can be categorized according to its severity in the following states [16]:

- The "*probable sarcopenia*" stage is characterized by low muscle strength with no effects on muscle mass or physical performance [16].

- The "*possible sarcopenia*" stage is characterized by low muscle strength or poor physical performance (normal muscle mass) [32].

- The "*presarcopenia*" stage is characterized by low muscle mass with no effects on muscle strength or physical performance [8].

- The "*sarcopenia*" stage is characterized by low muscle mass with low muscle strength or poor physical performance [8, 32, 33]. However, according to other authors this condition can also occur with low muscle mass and low muscle strength (without taking into account physical performance) or with low muscle mass and poor physical performance (without taking into account muscle strength) [13, 34].

- "Severe sarcopenia" or "severe" is the stage that is identified when the three parameters that determine sarcopenia are low: muscle mass, muscle strength, and physical performance [8, 16, 32].

Identifying the stages of sarcopenia helps in selecting treatments and setting appropriate recovery goals. Staging can also support the design of research studies that focus on a specific stage or changes in stages over time [8].

1.4 Parameters that define sarcopenia and variables that measure these parameters

The parameters that define sarcopenia are the amount of muscle and its function. The measurable variables are muscle mass, muscle strength, and physical performance [8].

Muscle mass can be expressed as total body skeletal muscle mass or as appendicular skeletal muscle mass, which is the sum of skeletal muscle mass of arms and legs [16].

Muscle strength refers to the amount of force that a muscle can produce with a single maximal effort [35].

The concept of the physical performance was defined for the first time to evaluate objectively and from a clinical point of view, how an individual performed different activities of daily living or physical tasks, as opposed to scales based on asking questions about the ability to perform these task [35]. However, since then, the concept of physical performance has evolved, and today, it is mainly related to ambulation and transfers [35], forming part of the most current definitions of sarcopenia.

The most up-to-date definition of physical performance was provided by Beaudart et al. [35] in 2019, who defined it as: "*A function of the whole body objectively related to locomotion*" (Beaudart et al., 2019).

1.5 Measurement of sarcopenia parameters

Currently, there are a wide variety of tests and tools available to measure the parameters that define sarcopenia [22, 36, 37], cost, availability, and ease of use, determine whether they are better adapted for clinical practice or more useful for research [8].

The selection of tools may depend on the patient (disability, mobility), access to technical resources in the setting where the tests are performed (community, clinic, hospital, or research center), or the purpose of the tests (monitoring of progression or follow-up of rehabilitation and recovery) [16].

Accurate measurement of muscle mass is a fundamental step to detect cases of patients with sarcopenia, and various techniques can be used for its quantification, but choosing one of them is not easy since all existing methods have advantages and disadvantages [38].

Nuclear magnetic resonance, computerized axial tomography, dual-energy X-ray absorptiometry, bioelectrical impedance analysis, determination of urinary creatinine excretion, and anthropometry are available [19].

There are few well-validated techniques to measure muscle strength, some assess upper extremity strength, and others lower extremity, and although the latter are more important for gait and physical function, and the two have been shown to be highly correlated [35]. Again, cost, availability, and ease of use determine whether techniques are best suited for clinical practice or useful for research purposes [8].

For the assessment of physical performance, there are a wide variety of tests. Short-distance walking tests can be used, such as the 2.4, 4, 6 m, or up to 10 m, or long-distance walking tests such as the 400-meter walk test, or the 6-minute walk test.

Other tests of physical performance are also the time up and go test (TUG), and the short physical performance battery (SPPB) [23].

2. Prevalence of sarcopenia according to the method used to determine physical performance

2.1 Prevalence of low physical performance

In the same definition of sarcopenia suggested by the European working group of Cruz-Jentoft et al. in 2010 (EWGSOP) [8], the prevalence of sarcopenia is already expected to be highly dependent on the method used to measure the diagnostic parameters of this disease and although there are several studies that have used the model proposed by the EWGSOP to determine the prevalence of sarcopenia and at least one from Beaudart et al. from 2015 [39], in which, using two different methods for both muscle mass and strength determination, significant differences were found in the prevalence of sarcopenia, as far as it has been found only the study of Sáez et al. de 2020 [40] compared the prevalence of sarcopenia, using three different methods for assessing physical performance, the usual gain speed (UGS), the time up and go test (TUG), and the short physical performance battery (SPPB), with the cut-off points recommended by the EWGSOP (**Table 1**).

According to this study, the prevalence of a low level of physical performance evaluated by these three different measurement methods, ranged globally, between 20.9 and 45.9%, increasing to 68.8% in the case of women [40]. The highest prevalence of low physical performance was obtained when evaluated by the UGS test, and it was lower for the TUG test (**Figure 2**). The prevalence of low physical performance was always higher in women than in men for any of the methods used for its determination [41]. These results are consistent with the fact that the average results of all physical performance tests were also lower for women [40].

Regarding the association and the concordance between the three tests used to assess physical performance, a significant association was found for all of them, with a low concordance, the overall concordance being between 71.1 and 78.6% [41]. These results show that the three tests used to determine physical performance are not interchangeable with each other and that the choice of one or the other would give significantly different results in the prevalence of physical performance [40].

2.2 Prevalence sarcopenia

According to these results of the study by Sáez et al. [40] that show a discordance in the prevalence of physical performance, and while this parameter is used for the diagnosis of sarcopenia, in the same way, we could expect discordant results on the prevalence of sarcopenia depending on the method used to determine physical performance, even applying the same diagnostic algorithm for all of them and defining sarcopenia as low muscle mass and low muscle function (muscle strength or physical performance) (**Table 2**) [8].

However, the results found showed similar sarcopenia prevalence values regardless of the method used for physical performance (6.0 vs. 63.9 vs. 67.0%) (**Table 3**) and with a concordance almost perfect [40].

Physical performance test	Cut points
Usual gain speed test (UGS)	≤0.8 m/s
Short physical performance battery (SPPB)	≤8 points
Up-and-go test (TUG)	≥20 seconds

Table 1.
Physical performance tests and cut points recommended by the EWGSOP.

Prevalence of physical performance measured by three different methods

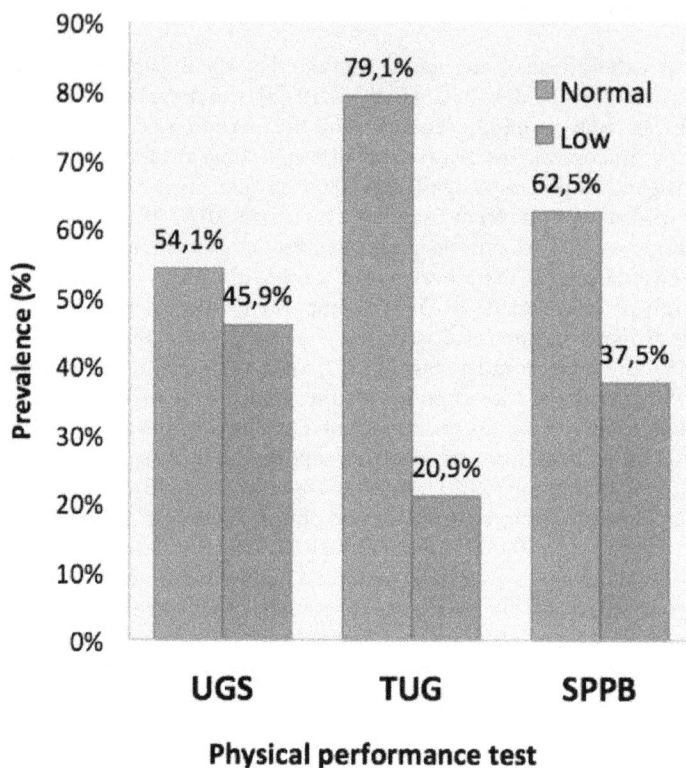

Figure 2.
Prevalence of physical performance using three different methods: Usual gait speed (UGS); get-up-go test (TUG); short physical performance battery (SPPB) (Sáez et al., 2020).

Muscle mass		Muscle function	
⇩	AND	Muscle straight	⇩
		OR	
		Physical performance	

Table 2.
Criteria for the diagnosis of sarcopenia according to the EWGSOP.

Physical performance test	Prevalence of sarcopenia		
	Total (%)	Men (%)	Women (%)
Usual gain speed test (UGS)	66.0	55.2	70.6
Short physical performance battery (SPPB)	63.9	55.2	67.6
Up-and-go test (TUG)	67.0	55.2	72.1

Table 3.
Sarcopenia prevalence comparing three different methods for the determination of physical performance (Sáez et al., 2020).

That is, an excellent concordance was found between the prevalence of sarcopenia regardless of the method used to assess physical performance, but at the same time with low concordance between the methods used to determine this parameter [40].

This finding allows us to hypothesize that possibly the diagnostic model used could not be dependent on the method used to determine physical performance and that therefore, the choice of one or another measurement technique for this parameter would not affect or influence the prevalence and the final diagnosis of sarcopenia [41].

These prevalence results are what would be expected and would be consistent with the definition of Cruz-Jentoft et al. of 2010 [8], suggesting that it is possible to choose any of the three methods of physical performance proposed by this group, which should be equally valid, and therefore give similar results for the prevalence of sarcopenia.

However, at this point, the following reflection could be made: *How is it possible that there is a significant difference in the prevalence of physical performance depending on the method chosen and a low concordance between the three methods used for its determination, and that the prevalence of sarcopenia has a near-perfect match? Could it be that physical performance was not a determining parameter for the diagnosis of sarcopenia?*

To answer these questions, it was proposed to apply a new model (**Table 4**), defining sarcopenia as low muscle strength plus low muscle mass and without taking physical performance into account, and comparing and assessing the concordance of the prevalence between this new algorithm and the one proposed by the EWGSOP in 2010 [40] for three different methods of assessing physical performance.

The prevalence of sarcopenia found according to this new algorithm was 63.9%, the association with the previous results, where physical performance was taken into account, was significant, and the agreement between them was excellent (**Figure 3**) [41].

These findings would indicate that indeed, being the agreement between the four cases almost perfect, physical performance does not seem to be determining or necessary for the diagnosis of sarcopenia [41].

The justification for these results is that for at least 95.4% of the cases in which the diagnosis is sarcopenia, muscle mass and strength have a low value, and according to the definition used for the diagnosis of sarcopenia (**Table 2**), this condition would be sufficient to confirm a positive case. In this way, the value, whether normal or low, of physical performance would no longer change the result of the diagnosis, and therefore for this 95.4% of cases, the method used to determine this parameter would no longer be relevant.

That is, most of the patients with low values of physical performance for any of the three tests (more than 82.4%) also had low values of muscle mass and strength [41], and thus when determining sarcopenia, the assessment of physical performance was indifferent.

Therefore, if the objectives were to find sarcopenia cases in a chosen population, a new diagnostic model, where sarcopenia was defined only by a low value of muscle strength plus a low value of muscle mass without having to assess physical performance [40], would be sufficient, to obtain the same results as with the model proposed by Cruz-Jentoft et al. in 2010 [8] where physical performance was taken into account.

The results found are also consistent and could in this way reinforce the proposal made by other authors such as Studenski et al. in 2014 [14] or Cruz-Jentoft et al. in 2019 [16] who proposed new diagnostic models, where sarcopenia was defined and

Muscle mass		Muscle straight
⇓	AND	⇓

Table 4.
New criteria proposal for the diagnosis of sarcopenia (Sáez et al., 2020).

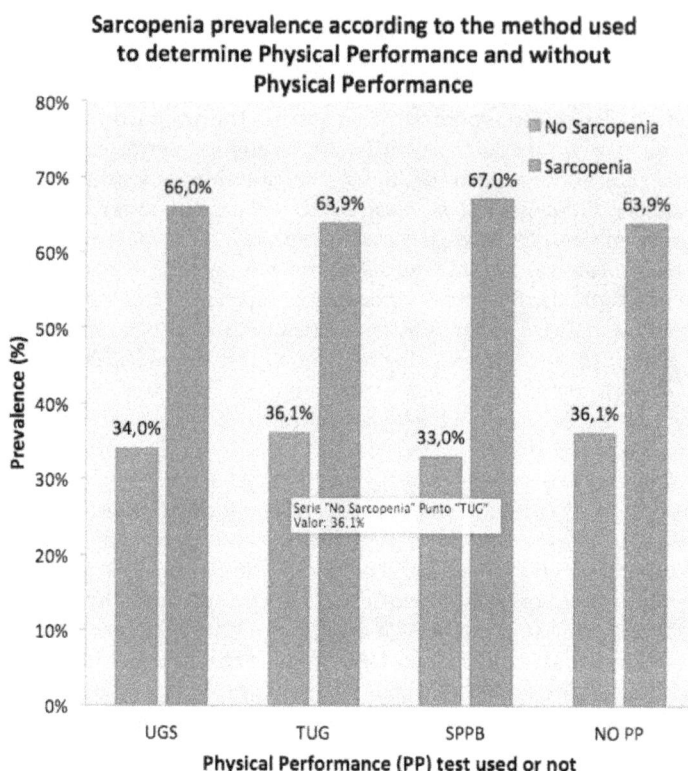

Figure 3.
Prevalence of sarcopenia using three different methods: Usual gait speed (UGS); get-up-go test (TUG); short physical performance battery (SPPB) and without physical performance (Sáez et al., 2020).

determined only taking into account these two properties of the muscle (strength and mass), without taking into account physical performance.

2.2.1 Older than 80 years

When the prevalence of sarcopenia was analyzed according to these four options, three taking into account physical performance and another without taking it into account, but for patients over 80 years of age, the results were even more conclusive, since the prevalence was the same in all cases (73.2%) and the agreement between them was perfect [41].

These results could mean two important things, first that sarcopenia is highly prevalent among the population over 65 years of age [42], but it could also mean that by increasing the age range from which sarcopenia is assessed, and the differences in the prevalence of this disease are reduced until identical results are found regardless of the method which is chosen to assess physical performance. This statement is consistent with that of other authors such as Petermann-Rocha et al. [43] who in a 2019 study in which they compared the prevalence between two diagnostic models, stated that the differences between the different results found in prevalence also decreased with increasing the age range considered. In other words, the greater the age range of the population studied, the less relevant it is to measure physical performance for the detection of cases of sarcopenia.

It has been found that concordance between these two diagnostic models remains perfect for patients 77 years of age or older and excellent for patients 75 years of age or older [41].

2.2.2 Sarcopenia staging

If the staging of sarcopenia in its different categories is taken into account (presarcopenia, sarcopenia, or severe sarcopenia), according to the model proposed by the EWGSOP in 2010, the results show that the prevalence of the state of presarcopenia and sarcopenia was higher for the physical performance measured with the TUG test, but for the severe sarcopenia state, the prevalence is higher with the UGS test [41].

Regarding the prevalence of absence of sarcopenia, it is observed that it is the same regardless of the method used for physical performance [41]. This is consistent since according to the EWGSOP definition, the absence of sarcopenia is determined only by a normal value of muscle mass, regardless of the value of the other two diagnostic parameters.

Regarding the association and concordance between the prevalence of sarcopenia states according to the method used for physical performance, a significant association was found and a global concordance percentage was greater than 76.0% in all cases, being the best 86.6% between the TUG and SPPB tests [41].

As mentioned above, a low concordance was found between the methods used to assess physical performance, and although on the other hand, it seems that the prevalence of sarcopenia would be independent of the method used to assess physical performance when assessing sarcopenia according to its states, it is observed that, although for the case of absence of sarcopenia, there are no variations in prevalence (17.5% for the three methods), for the state of presarcopenia, the greatest variation was 3.1% between the TUG test and the SPPB test, but these differences increased up to 16.5% points for the case of the severe sarcopenia state, between the UGS test and the TUG test [41]. The TUG test is the one that shows the greatest difference with respect to the other two in both sarcopenia and severe sarcopenia states.

These differences are due, on the one hand, to the fact that, as already mentioned, the three physical performance tests are not concordant with each other, and although it was found that this aspect did not influence the prevalence of sarcopenia, however, the severity of sarcopenia is influenced by physical performance, since according to the EWGSOP definition, the three diagnostic parameters must be low (**Table 2**).

When the prevalence of a low value of physical performance was assessed, precisely the TUG test was the one with the lowest prevalence (20.9%) with a difference of 25.0% points compared to the UGS test and 16.6% points regarding the SPPB, which is why the lowest value of severe sarcopenia was also obtained with this test [41].

On the other hand, it was the UGS test that had the highest prevalence of a low value for physical performance, which is why it was also the test that obtained the highest prevalence of severe sarcopenia. In fact, the higher the prevalence of the low value of physical performance, the higher the prevalence of severe sarcopenia [41].

This result was consistent with the definition of severe sarcopenia, for which this state only occurred with the low values of the three diagnostic parameters of this disease (**Table 2**), and therefore, physical performance is a necessary parameter if we want to determine the severity of sarcopenia.

3. Conclusions

The prevalence of sarcopenia obtained by applying the diagnostic algorithm proposed by the EWGSOP in 2010 [8] was very similar regardless of the method, which was used to determine physical performance. However, we also found that the prevalence of poor physical performance was dependent on the method used to measure it. The apparent incongruity between these two conclusions could be explained by a third; that is, physical performance might not be a necessary parameter for the diagnosis of sarcopenia and therefore, it might be sufficient to use a simplified diagnostic algorithm that takes into account only strength and muscle mass but not the physical performance and obtain the same diagnostic results for sarcopenia. Finally, we conclude that the results found are consistent and reinforce the proposal made by the EWGSOP in 2018 [16] where physical performance is no longer a necessary parameter for determining sarcopenia, although it could be to determine the severity of this disease.

Conflict of interest

The authors declare no conflict of interest.

Nomenclature

EWGSOP	European Working Group on Sarcopenia in Older People
ICD	International Classification of Diseases
TUG	timed up-and-go
UGS	usual gain speed
SPPB	short physical performance battery

Author details

Carlos Sáez* and Sara García-Isidoro
Pontifical University of Salamanca, Madrid, Spain

*Address all correspondence to: jcgordillosa@upsa.es

IntechOpen

References

[1] Rosenberg IH. Sarcopenia: Origins and clinical relevance. The Journal of Nutrition. 1997;**127**(5):990S-991S

[2] Pomeransky AA, Khriplovich IB, Rosenberg IH. Summary comments: Epidemiological and methodological problems in determining nutritional status of older persons. The American Journal of Clinical Nutrition. 1989;**50**(1-3):145-173

[3] Delmonico MJ, Harris TB, Visser M, Park SW, Conroy MB, Velasquez-Mieyer P, et al. Longitudinal study of muscle strength, quality, and adipose tissue infiltration. The American Journal of Clinical Nutrition. 2009;**90**(5):1579-1585

[4] M McLean RR, Kiel DP. Developing consensus criteria for sarcopenia: An update. J Bone Miner Res. 2015 Apr;**30**(4):588-592. DOI: 10.1002/jbmr.2492.

[5] Morley JE, Baumgartner RN, Roubenoff R, Mayer J, Nair KS. Sarcopenia. The Journal of Laboratory and Clinical Medicine. 2001;**137**(4):231-243

[6] Cooper C, Dere W, Evans W, Kanis JA, Rizzoli R, Sayer AA, et al. Frailty and sarcopenia: Definitions and outcome parameters. Osteoporosis International. 2012;**23**(7):1839-1848

[7] Newman AB, Kupelian V, Visser M, Simonsick E, Goodpaster B, Nevitt M, et al. Sarcopenia: Alternative definitions and associations with lower extremity function. Journal of the American Geriatrics Society. 2003;**51**(11):1602-1609

[8] Cruz-Jentoft A, Baeyens JP, Bauer JM, Boirie Y, Cederholm T, Landi F, et al. Sarcopenia: European consensus on definition and diagnosis: Report of the European Working Group

on sarcopenia in older people. Age and Ageing. 2010;**39**(4):412-423

[9] Beaudart C, McCloskey E, Bruyère O, Cesari M, Rolland Y, Rizzoli R, et al. Sarcopenia in daily practice: Assessment and management. BMC Geriatrics. 2016;**16**(1):170

[10] Ethgen O, Beaudart C, Buckinx F, Bruyère O, Reginster JY. The future prevalence of sarcopenia in Europe: A claim for public health action. Calcified Tissue International. 2017;**100**(3):229-234

[11] Falcon LJ, Harris-Love MO. Sarcopenia and the new ICD-10-CM code: Screening, staging, and diagnosis considerations. Federal Practitioner. 2017;**34**(7):24-32

[12] Cao L, Morley JE. Sarcopenia is recognized as an independent condition by an International Classification of Disease, Tenth Revision, Clinical Modification (ICD-10-CM) Code. Journal of the American Medical Directors Association. 2016;**17**(8):675-677

[13] Morley JE, Abbatecola AM, Argiles JM, Baracos V, Bauer J, Bhasin S, et al. Sarcopenia with limited mobility: An international consensus. Journal of the American Medical Directors Association. 2011;**12**(6):403-409

[14] Studenski SA, Peters KW, Alley DE, Cawthon PM, McLean RR, Harris TB, et al. The FNIH sarcopenia project: Rationale, study description, conference recommendations, and final estimates. Journals of Gerontology, Series A. 2014;**69**(5):547-558

[15] Bone AE, Hepgul N, Kon S, Maddocks M. Sarcopenia and frailty in chronic respiratory disease. Chronic Respiratory Disease. 2017;**14**(1):85-99

[16] Cruz-Jentoft A, Bahat G, Bauer J, Boirie Y, Bruyère O, Cederholm T, et al.

Sarcopenia: Revised European consensus on definition and diagnosis. Age and Ageing. 2019;**48**(1):16-31

[17] Di Monaco M, Vallero F, Di Monaco R, Tappero R. Prevalence of sarcopenia and its association with osteoporosis in 313 older women following a hip fracture. Archives of Gerontology and Geriatrics. 2011; **52**(1):71-74

[18] Lauretani F, Russo CR, Bandinelli S, Bartali B, Cavazzini C, Di Iorio A, et al. Age-associated changes in skeletal muscles and their effect on mobility: An operational diagnosis of sarcopenia. Journal of Applied Physiology. 2003;**95**(5):1851-1860

[19] Rolland Y, Czerwinski S, Van Kan GA, Morley JE, Cesari M, Onder G, et al. Sarcopenia: Its assessment, etiology, pathogenesis, consequences and future perspectives. The Journal of Nutrition, Health & Aging. 2008;**12**(7): 433-450

[20] Delmonico MJ, Harris TB, Lee J-S, Visser M, Nevitt M, Kritchevsky SB, et al. Alternative definitions of sarcopenia, lower extremity performance, and functional impairment with aging in older men and women. Journal of the American Geriatrics Society. 2007;**55**(5):769-774

[21] Goodpaster BH, Park SW, Harris TB, Kritchevsky SB, Nevitt M, Schwartz AV, et al. The loss of skeletal muscle strength, mass, and quality in older adults: The health, aging and body composition study. The Journals of Gerontology. Series A, Biological Sciences and Medical Sciences. 2006;**61**(10):1059-1064

[22] Bruyère O, Beaudart C, Reginster J-Y, Buckinx F, Schoene D, Hirani V, et al. Assessment of muscle mass, muscle strength and physical performance in clinical practice: An international survey. European Geriatric Medicine. 2016;**7**(3):243-246

[23] Kim KM, Jang HC, Lim S. Differences among skeletal muscle mass indices derived from height-, weight-, and body mass index-adjusted models in assessing sarcopenia. The Korean Journal of Internal Medicine. 2016;**31**(4):643-650

[24] Beaudart C, Zaaria M, Pasleau FF, Reginster J-YY, Bruyère O. Health outcomes of sarcopenia: A systematic review and meta-analysis. PLoS One. 2017;**12**(1):1-16

[25] Beaudart C, Reginster JY, Petermans J, Gillain S, Quabron A, Locquet M, et al. Quality of life and physical components linked to sarcopenia: The SarcoPhAge study. Experimental Gerontology. 2015;**69**:103-110

[26] Bischoff-Ferrari HA, Orav JE, Kanis JA, Rizzoli R, Schlögl M, Staehelin HB, et al. Comparative performance of current definitions of sarcopenia against the prospective incidence of falls among community-dwelling seniors age 65 and older. Osteoporosis International. 2015;**26**(12):2793-2802

[27] Schaap LA, van Schoor NM, Lips P, Visser M. Associations of sarcopenia definitions, and their components, with the incidence of recurrent falling and fractures: The longitudinal aging study Amsterdam. Journals of Gerontology, Series A. 2018;**73**(9):1199-1204

[28] Malmstrom TK, Miller DK, Simonsick EM, Ferrucci L, Morley JE. SARC-F: A symptom score to predict persons with sarcopenia at risk for poor functional outcomes. Journal of Cachexia, Sarcopenia and Muscle. 2016;**7**(1):28-36

[29] Bahat G, İlhan B. Sarcopenia and the cardiometabolic syndrome: A narrative review. European Geriatric Medicine. 2016;**7**(3):220-223

[30] Chang KV, Hsu TH, Wu WT, Huang KC, Han DS. Association between sarcopenia and cognitive impairment: A systematic review and meta-analysis. Journal of the American Medical Directors Association. 2016;**17**(12):1164.e7-1164.e15

[31] Beaudart C, Biver E, Reginster J-YY, Rizzoli R, Rolland Y, Bautmans I, et al. Validation of the SarQoL®, a specific health-related quality of life questionnaire for sarcopenia. Journal of Cachexia, Sarcopenia and Muscle. 2017;**8**(2):238-244

[32] Chen L-K, Woo J, Assantachai P, Auyeung T-W, Chou M-Y, Iijima K, et al. Asian working group for sarcopenia: 2019 consensus update on sarcopenia diagnosis and treatment. Journal of the American Medical Directors Association. 2020;**21**(3):300-307.e2

[33] Chen L-K, Liu L-K, Woo J, Assantachai P, Auyeung T-W, Bahyah KS, et al. Sarcopenia in Asia: Consensus report of the Asian working group for sarcopenia. Journal of the American Medical Directors Association. 2014;**15**(2):95-101

[34] Fielding RA, Vellas B, Evans WJ, Bhasin S, Morley JE, Newman AB, et al. Sarcopenia: An undiagnosed condition in older adults. Current consensus definition: Prevalence, etiology, and consequences. International Working Group on Sarcopenia. Journal of the American Medical Directors Association. 2011;**12**(4):249-256

[35] Beaudart C, Rolland Y, Cruz-Jentoft AJ, Bauer JM, Sieber C, Cooper C, et al. Assessment of muscle function and physical performance in daily clinical practice. Calcified Tissue International. 2019;**105**(1):1-14

[36] Reginster J-Y, Cooper C, Rizzoli R, Kanis JA, Appelboom G, Bautmans I, et al. Recommendations for the conduct of clinical trials for drugs to treat or

prevent sarcopenia. Aging Clinical and Experimental Research. 2016;**28**(1): 47-58

[37] Mijnarends DM, Meijers JMMM, Halfens RJGG, Ter Borg S, Luiking YC, Verlaan S, et al. Validity and reliability of tools to measure muscle mass, strength, and physical performance in community-dwelling older people: A systematic review. Journal of the American Medical Directors Association. 2013;**14**(3):170-178

[38] Masanés Torán F, Navarro López M, Sacanella Meseguer E, López SA. ¿Qué es la sarcopenia? Seminarios de la Fundacion Espanola de Reumatologia. 2010;**11**(1):14-23

[39] Beaudart C, Reginster JY, Slomian J, Buckinx F, Dardenne N, Quabron A, et al. Estimation of sarcopenia prevalence using various assessment tools. Experimental Gerontology. 2015;**61**:31-37

[40] Sáez C, Delaire L, García-Isidoro S, De-la-Gala F, Bonnefoy M. Comparación de la prevalencia de sarcopenia en personas de edad avanzada según el algoritmo propuesto por el EWGSOP en 2010 para la identificación de casos de sarcopenia utilizando tres métodos diferentes para la determinación del rendimiento físico. Fisioterapia. 2020;**42**(3):115-123

[41] Sáez C, García-Isidoro S, De-la-Gala F. Sarcopenia, una condición sin consenso diagnóstico en la actualidad. Definiciones actuales y comparación entre los diferentes modelos diagnósticos propuestos por los principales grupos de trabajo internacionales sobre la sarcopenia en personas de edad avanzada. Potifical University of Salamanca; Dialnet. 2020. Available from: https://dialnet.unirioja.es/servlet/tesis?codigo=283413

[42] Landi F, Calvani R, Picca A, Tosato M, Bernabei R, Marzetti E.

Emerging research on importance of muscle mass and function. Journal of Gerontology and Geriatrics. 2019; **67**(1):26-31

[43] Petermann-Rocha F, Chen M, Gray SR, Ho FK, Pell JP, Celis-Morales C. New versus old guidelines for sarcopenia classification: What is the impact on prevalence and health outcomes? Age and Ageing. 2019;**49**(2):300-304

Sarcopenia in Patients with End-Stage Cardiac Failure Requiring Ventricular Assist Device or Heart Transplantation

Norihide Fukushima

Abstract

Sarcopenia has been defined as the age-related reduced skeletal muscle mass, strength, and physical capacity and is frequently associated with serious complications in patients with heart failure (HF). However, when HF progressed to end-stage HF requiring advanced therapies, such as heart transplantation (HTx) and implantation of left ventricular assist device (LVAD), an even higher prevalence of sarcopenia has been reported in younger patients with end-stage HF than elderly patients with less advanced HF. Many literatures have reported that sarcopenia is greatly associated with high rates of morbidity and mortality after HTx and LVAD implantation. Therefore, therapeutic interventions to prevent and reverse sarcopenia, such as cardiac rehabilitation and nutrition supplementation, are important in patients with end-stage HF prior to HTx and LVAD implantation. Although moderate or severe sarcopenia is a contraindication for HTx, the patients who can recover from sarcopenia after LVAD implantation would be considered eligible for HTx. Then, therapeutic options to reverse sarcopenia in patients supported with LVAD are also important to improve patient prognosis after LVAD implantation. In this review, the impacts of sarcopenia on prognosis after LVAD implantation and HTx and vice versa were summarized and therapeutic interventions to reverse sarcopenia before and after LVAD implantation are discussed.

Keywords: sarcopenia, end-stage heart failure, heart transplantation, left ventricular assist device, cardiac rehabilitation, nutrition supplementation

1. Introduction

Heart failure (HF) is a general acute and chronic disease expressing the advanced stage of various types of heart disease, and its prevalence is increasing year by year [1]. As the risk of HF increases with age [2], elderly patients occupy more than four-fifth of all patients with HF. HF may reduce organ and physical functional capacity and their daily life performance in patients. HF greatly affects physical function as well as body composition of skeletal muscle, which is greatly correlated with high rates of morbidity, hospitalization, and mortality [3, 4].

Sarcopenia is a syndrome characterized by general skeletal muscle mass loss and strength, which is related to poor outcomes and high mortality in patients with a variety of underlying diseases [5]. Although sarcopenia has been first defined as an age-related syndrome, it was also frequently associated with serious complications in even younger patients with advanced stage of HF [6, 7]. The alteration in the skeletal muscle system in patients with HF plays the main role in developing many signs and symptoms related to HF [8, 9]. Then, sarcopenia may significantly greatly attribute to the poor prognosis in patients with HF than in those of the same age without HF [8]. The rate of sarcopenia in a patient with HF is reported to be higher at 19.5% than that in healthy individuals of the same age [10]. Although sarcopenia is more frequently associated with increasing age, an even higher prevalence of 47% has been reported in patients younger than 55 years with dilated cardiomyopathy [11]. Therefore, the patient population with end-stage HF requiring ventricular assist device (VAD) or heart transplantation (HTx) may be different from those with less advanced HF.

Even in younger patients with end-stage HF, metabolic abnormalities related to sarcopenia develop and affect renal and hepatic function [11]. Skeletal muscle, which is the greatest reservoir of protein, is easily wasted in catabolic illness including end-stage HF. However, therapeutic interventions to reverse progressive local and systemic catabolism in advanced HF are limited. Growth hormone (GH) administration and aerobic exercise rehabilitation are known to increase insulin-like growth factor (IGF)-1 level in the blood and increase skeletal muscle volume in HF [12–14]. VAD implantation for bridge-to-transplantation (BTT) and destination therapy (DT) improves local and systemic metabolism probably due to corrected hemodynamics and tissue perfusion in patients with end-stage HF [15, 16]. Multiple literatures have reported that advanced strategies for HF, such as VAD implantation and HTx, provide optimal hemodynamic support and improve local and systemic metabolism, resulting in improvement of other organ function as well as physical capacity [17, 18].

Due to the great development in the field of left VAD (LVAD) in the past two decades, patients referred to this therapy are greatly increased. Although great advances in methodology and increased clinical experience in LVAD therapy had improved patient survival with end-stage HF over time, a certain amount of patients still has a high prevalence of mortality, comorbidity, and hospitalization after LVAD implantation, even in clinical trial settings [19]. As patients for DT are older and have more commodities before LVAD implantation than those for BTT, the use of LVAD for DT recently approved clinically worldwide may lead to higher mortality and morbidity in patients implanted with LVAD.

In this article, we review the impacts of both VAD and HTx on variables associated with sarcopenia as well as malnutrition in patients with end-stage HF and vice versa and discuss therapeutic interventions to reverse sarcopenia before and after LVAD implantation.

2. Diagnosis of sarcopenia

According to the consensus on definition and diagnosis by the European Working Group on Sarcopenia in Older People (EWGSOP), sarcopenia is defined by the presence of both reduced skeletal muscle mass and function as well as reduced physical performance (**Figure 1**) [20]. Skeletal muscle strength is assessed by handgrip strength (HGS), whereas physical performance is assessed by usual gait speed. In the presence of reduced skeletal muscle function, defined by a reduced gait speed (<0.8 m/s) and/or a reduced HGS (<26–30 kg for men and <16–20 kg for women), the diagnosis requires verification of reduced skeletal muscle mass. Currently, magnetic resonance imaging (MRI) and computed tomography (CT)

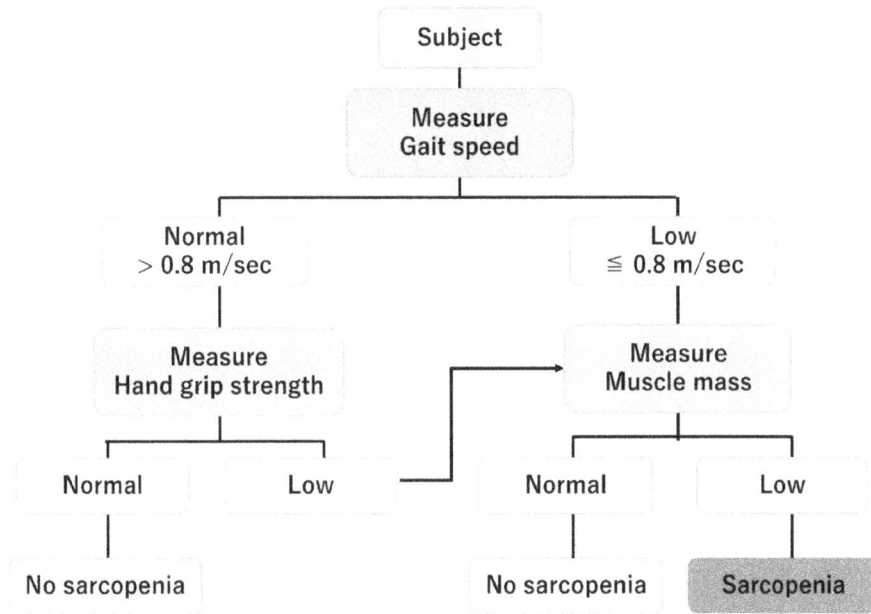

Figure 1.
Sarcopenia assessment algorithm.

have been the gold standard to accurately measure the mass of a skeletal muscle as well as its density and fatty infiltration.

The HGS is an easy and simple tool but suffers from that peripheral muscle strength and function might improve after LVAD implantation and HTx as previously described [21, 22]. To resolve these limitations, investigators in the field of mechanical circulatory support and HTx have begun to estimate the grade of sarcopenia by evaluating the mass of skeletal muscles, such as psoas and pectoralis muscles with clinical prognosis. Positive results have been reported in patients undergoing invasive thoracic and abdominal surgeries [23–26] as well as in those with advanced HF [27–29]. CT scans provide precise identification and quantification of individual skeletal muscle and fat tissue components [30–32].

Creatinine excretion rate index (CER index) in 24-hour urine collection is an easily measurable and less invasive classic marker of total-body skeletal muscle mass [33] and a reliable biomarker even in patients with advanced HF [34, 35]. Iwasaki et al. [36] reported that the CER index in patients with continuous-flow implantable LVAD (CF-LVAD) was significantly correlated with psoas and pectoralis muscles mass measured by CT scan.

3. Impact of sarcopenia at pre-LVAD on outcome after LVAD implantation

Clinical studies of sarcopenia in patients with advanced heart failure referred for left ventricular assist device implantation or heart transplantation is summarized in (**Table 1**).

3.1 Skeletal muscle function

Chung et al. [21] examined the correlation of HGS with outcomes after LVAD implantation, showing that HGS less than 25% of body weight was related to higher

Study	Population	No.	Mean age (years) Gender	Sarcopenia assessment	Main findings	Comment
Chung [21]	Pre- and post LVAD	72	59 89% male	Reduced HGS < 25% body weight	HGS < 25% at pre-LVAD associated with increased operative mortality and postoperative complications. HGS increased by 18.2 +/- 5.6% at 3 months (n 5 29) and 45.5 +/- 23.9% at 6 months post-LVAD implantation.	Reduced HGS in 22% pre-LVAD Improved HGS in survivors at 3 and 6 months post-LVAD. HGS correlated with serum albumin level. HGS was measured with Jamar dynamometer.
Khawaja [22]	Pre-BTT LVAD	25	62 88% male	HGS	Mean HGS at pre-LVAD 35.8 +/- 7.8 vs. 55.6 +/- 12.7 kg in control (no cardiac disease, nonsmokers) (P < 0.05) % increase in HGS at 6 mo on LVAD: +26.5 +/- 27.5% (P = 0.05)	LVAD implantation corrects GH/IGF-1 signaling, improves muscle structure and function, and enhances oxidative muscle metabolism in patients with advanced HF
Heberton [37]	Pre-DT LVAD	100	54 77% male	Psoas muscle area on CT scan at L3-L4 level defined as lowest tertile for gender	Significant increase in composite endpoint of prolonged hospital-stay or inpatient mortality (P = 0.043)	Retrospective study 100 of 333 patients with usable CT scans The psoas muscle area cut-off values for the lowest tertiles were 12.0 cm² for men and 6.5 cm² for women, resulting in 32 sarcopenic patients (32%).
Teigen [32]	Pre-BTT LVAD	143	60 89% male	PMI and PHUm pre-LVAD	Increased PMI and PHUm associated with a 27% reduction in the hazard of death after LVAD	For PMI, the estimated survival by tertile was the following: highest 86%, middle 84%, and lowest 59% (P = 0.002 by log-rank test).
Fernandes [38]	Pre-HTx (on Waiting list)	23	51 87% male	CSAbPm, HGS, MIP and MEP in waiting list group and after HTx	Reduced CSAbPm, HGS, MIP and MEP in waiting list group compared to healthy control Increased CSAbPm, HGS, MIP and MEP in patients surviving longer than 6 mo after HTx	

Study	Population	No.	Mean age (years) Gender	Sarcopenia assessment	Main findings	Comment
Cogswell [39]	Pre-BTT LVAD	Not defined	Not defined	Minnesota Pectoralis Risk Score (MPRS),	The calculated MPRS place each patient in the low, medium, or high-risk category and estimates survival probability at 30, 60, and 365 days after LVAD implantation.	MPRS was calculated by a set of predictors, such as a PHUm, PMI, African American race, creatinine, total bilirubin, body mass index, bridge to transplant, and the presence or absence of contrast. Receiver-operating characteristic curves for 30-, 90-, and 365-day survival were generated. The area under the curve for the model at 30, 90, and 365 days was 0.78, 0.76, and 0.76, respectively.
Tsuji [40]	Pre-BTT LVAD	78	42 71% male	Skeletal muscle index (SMI) on CT scan at L3 level	Muscle wasting was associated with post-LVAD mortality (hazard ratio: 4.32; 95% CI: 1.19–20.2)	The SMI cut-off values for the lowest tertiles were 36.7 cm^2/m^2 for men and 28.2 cm^2/m^2 for women, resulting in 26 patients (33.3%) with muscle wasting.
Iwasaki [36]	Pre-BTT LVAD	147	44 72% male	Creatinine excretion rate (CER) index	A low CER index was an independent predictor of intracranial hemorrhage in patients receiving a CF-iLVAD	CER index = [Cr]urine×24-h urine volume/body weight
Cogswell [41]	Pre-LVAD	276	61 84% male	PMI	Patients in the low PMI group associated with post-LVAD mortality irrespectively of INTERMACS profile, but INTERMACS 3 and 4 patients in the high PMI groups had the highest survival on LVAD support	Patients with the largest deterioration in renal function (highest slope) between −365 and −60 days before LVAD were more likely to be INTERMACS 1 and 2 at the time of LVAD implantation.

Abbreviations: LVAD left ventricular assist device, HGS handgrip strength, BTT bridge to transplant,, GH: growth hormone, IGF-1: insulin-like growth factor, DT destination therapy, CT computed tomography, PMI Unilateral Pectoralis muscle mass indexed to BSA, PHUm pectoralis muscle mean Hounsfield unit, HTx: heart transplantation, CSAbPm cross-sectional area of the bilateral psoas major muscle, MIP and MEP the maximum inspiratory and expiratory pressure body surface area, CI confidence interval, Cr serum creatinine.

Table 1.
Clinical studies of sarcopenia in patients with advanced heart failure referred for left ventricular assist device implantation or heart transplantation.

mortality. Khawaja et al. [22] reported that patients with advanced HF had significantly lower HGS prior to CF-LVAD implantation compared to healthy controls and that the average HGS increased greater than 25% after 6 months after CF-LVAD implantation.

3.2 Skeletal muscle mass measurement

Heberton et al. [37] first introduced the assessment of skeletal muscle mass in the field of LVAD therapy and reported that sarcopenia by measuring psoas muscle area at L3-L4 vertebrae was significantly related to longer hospital stay and higher mortality after implantation of HeartMate II LVAD. On the other hand, Teigen et al. reported that pectoralis muscle mass and tissue quality by measuring Hounsfield units (PHUm) and size-indexed to body surface area were highly associated with post-LVAD mortality and surpassed any other variables in the University of Minnesota dataset [32]. This group further added an external dataset to create a user-friendly, multivariable post-LVAD mortality-prediction score, the so-called the Minnesota Pectoralis Risk Score (MPRS) [39]. This final model included PHUm, pectoralis muscle index (PMI), African American race, serum creatinine and total bilirubin, body mass index (BMI), BTT or DT, and the presence or absence of contrast. The estimated 1-year survival for patients after LVAD implantation by MPRS risk category (tertiles) was the following—low, medium, and high risks were 95, 79, and 58%, respectively (P < 0.0001 by log-rank test). These skeletal muscle measures appear to add important prognostic value to pre-LVAD risk assessment [39]. A further study by them [41] described that INTERMACS 3 and four patients with the highest PMI had the best survival after CF-LVAD implantation. Tsuji et al. [40] also reported that muscle wasting defined by skeletal muscle index on CT scan at L3 level was also associated with post-LVAD mortality. From these findings, CT scan quantification of sarcopenia may help us to identify the optimal timing of LVAD implantation.

3.3 Creatinine excretion rate index

Iwasaki et al. [36] reported that reduced CER index was significantly related to a higher rate of mortality and intracranial hemorrhage after CF-LVAD implantation. Preoperative reduced CER index might be an independent predictor of intracranial hemorrhage after CF-LVAD implantation.

4. Impact of sarcopenia as well as malnutrition at pre-HTx on outcome after HTx

4.1 Sarcopenia and indication for HTx

The donor heart shortage restricts HTx to a small portion of potential recipients. Moreover, serious complications accompanied with patients with end-stage HF, such as sarcopenia, systemic infection, and irreversible renal and hepatic dysfunction, more greatly affect patient prognosis after HTx than other cardiac surgery, because HTx recipients need immunosuppressive medication to prevent allograft rejection. Therefore, HTx is a treatment option for a few carefully selected patients with end-stage HF. The number of patients above the age of 60 years being transplanted has increased over the past 10 years. And recent post-HTx survival in patients aged between 60 and 69 years has been satisfactory. However, 5-year mortality in those aged 70 years and older are significantly poorer compared with those aged between 18 and 59 years. Therefore, recipients aged older than 70 years are less acutely ill, have fewer comorbidities, and are less likely to have durable LVAD support for BTT [42]. Therefore, usually moderate or severe sarcopenia, as well as frailty, might be a contraindication for HTx. However, LVAD implantation in patients with frailty could be applicable as a bridge to candidacy. Patients who can recover from a frail state after LVAD implantation presumably after a certain period of physical rehabilitation and nutrition supplementation would then be considered eligible for HTx. This means that a sarcopenia patient who is firstly likely to survive LVAD implantation and secondly to reverse his/her frailty or sarcopenia can be a potential candidate for HTx [43]. For these reasons, there has been no published data concerning the impacts of real sarcopenia on outcomes after HTx.

4.2 Impact of malnutrition and physical rehabilitation at before and after HTx on exercise capacity post-HTx

Although previous studies have shown that the recipients exhibit improvements in exercise capacity and physical performance after HTx, the recipients often have a lower exercise capacity than normal healthy controls of the same age and gender soon and long after HTx.

Yanase et al. [44] investigated the effects of the recipient and donor predictive risk factors on the patient's exercise capacity early after HTx. In this study, 3-month rehabilitation exercise training significantly increased peak VO2 irrespective of the main recipient or donor risk predictive factors on post-HTx survival, which included paracorporeal or implantable LVAD, and several marginal donor heart risk factors. Only younger recipient age and better several nutrition factors, such as higher choline esterase and higher blood lymphocyte count, at the entry of 3-month exercise program were significantly associated with higher peak VO2 at the entry and the end of the 3-month training program. These data suggested that nutrition management and rehabilitation at the bedside prior to starting the exercise training program play a significant role in increasing peak VO2 at the entry of the rehabilitation program.

5. Impact of LVAD implantation on sarcopenia

As mentioned earlier, many investigators have shown that sarcopenia was associated with increased comorbidity and mortality after implantation of LVAD. On the other hand, only limited studies concerning the impact of LVAD implantation on sarcopenia have been available. Several investigators reported improvement of HGS after implantation of CF-LVAD [21, 22]. Although it has been reported that frailty prior to BTT LVAD implantation is associated with an increased post-LVAD morbidity and mortality, it has also been reported that frailty is reversible in most patients who survive the perioperative period [45, 46]. Maurer et al. [47] assessed reversal of frailty in 29 elderly frail LVAD recipients with a mean age of 71 years. Although frailty improved overall, 53% of the patients remained frail 6 months after LVAD implantation. These data suggested that frailty may be less reversible in aged patients supported with LVAD.

Multiple studies have shown that implantation of LVAD not only provides adequate hemodynamic support but also improves renal and liver function and psychical capacity especially after receiving physical rehabilitation. However, there are multifactorial limitations to exercise in patients supported with LVAD [38]. Although LVAD implantation improves hemodynamics in end-stage HF patients at rest, the device is unable to provide full circulatory support during exercise, especially in patients with CF-LVAD. Thus, significant limitations in exercise capacity persist soon and long after CF-LVAD implantation. Maximizing LV unloading and improving native myocardial function in association with an automated increase in LVAD speed could provide an increase in maximal exercise capacity in patients with the old-type pulsatile implantable LVAD. However, CF-LVAD can provide only partial improvement in maximal exercise capacity. Further studies are needed regarding the role of RV function, recovery of native cardiac function, the role of rehabilitation and nutrition intervention, changes in skeletal muscle function after CF-LVAD, and their contribution to endurance exercise [38].

6. Impact of HTx on sarcopenia

Fernandes et al. [48] investigated the impact of HTx on the recovery of peripheral and respiratory muscle mass and strength in patients with congestive HF. They showed significant decreases in a cross-sectional area of the bilateral psoas major muscle (CSAbPm), a bilateral HGS, and the maximum inspiratory and expiratory pressure (MIP and MEP) in patients on the waiting list compared with the healthy controls with normal cardiac function. They also found significant increases during waiting for HTx to 6- and 18-month post-HTx in the CSAbPm (1305.4 vs. 1458.1 vs. 1431.3 mm^2, respectively), bilateral HGS (27.3 vs. 30.2 vs. 34.7 kg/f, respectively), MIP (59.5 vs. 85.5 vs. 90.9 cmH$_2$O, respectively), and MEP (79.5 vs. 93.2 vs. 101.8 cmH$_2$O, respectively). These results revealed that patients recovered peripheral and respiratory muscle mass and strength early after HTx. However, Schaufelberger et al. [49] demonstrated that intrinsic abnormalities in skeletal muscle found before HTx remained 6–9 months after HTx and might contribute to a reduced exercise capacity and muscle strength in these patients, in contrast to the former paper's findings.

7. Management of sarcopenia after LVAD implantation

As mentioned earlier, sarcopenia is a strong negative predictor on outcome after LVAD implantation and HTx. Therefore, sarcopenia is one of the main therapeutic targets in patients with end-stage HF referred to LVAD implantation and HTx to avoid related comorbidity and to improve prognosis post-LVAD implantation and post-HTx. Although moderate or severe sarcopenia as well as frailty is a contraindication for HTx, patients who can reverse frail after LVAD implantation would be considered eligible for HTx. Therefore, to further improve outcomes after LVAD implantation or HTx, therapeutic management for sarcopenia should be established in patients supported with LVAD as well as those prior to LVAD implantation. As the management of sarcopenia in patients prior to LVAD implantation might be the same in medically treated patients with end-stage HF and has been previously well discussed in many previous literatures, those for patients supported with CF-LVAD will be discussed in this review.

According to the pathophysiological factors involved in the pathogenesis of sarcopenia, therapeutic approaches for sarcopenia are summarized in **Figure 2**. Although Khawaja et al. [22] reported that CF-LVAD implantation corrects GH/IGF-1 signaling and improves muscle structure and function, only limited data were available regarding anti-inflammation strategies and hormonal therapies, such as GF/IGF-1 and ghrelin administration for sarcopenia in patients supported with LVAD. Therefore, exercise training and nutrition supplementation in patients supported with LVAD are reviewed in this review.

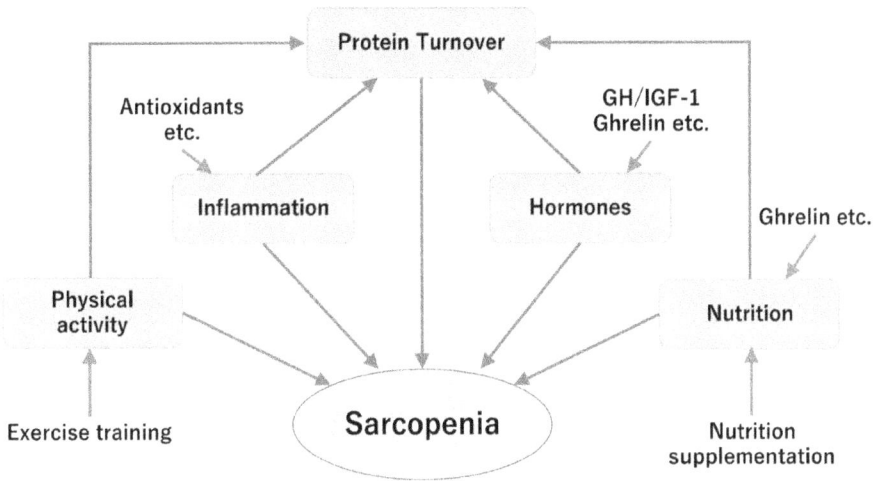

Figure 2.
Sarcopenia pathogenesis and therapeutic approaches: GH growth hormone, IGF-1 insulin-like growth factor-1.

7.1 Exercise training (rehabilitation) in LVAD patients

Generally, HTx or LVAD recipients attend a cardiac rehabilitation program to promote recovery after surgery. Such rehabilitation programs consist of standardized sessions of physical exercise training, with the same intensity and duration regardless of HTx or LVAD implantation. However, surgical indication and method, individual medical and surgical therapies, and possible adverse events after surgery might affect the efficacy of cardiac rehabilitation differently in HTx and LVAD patients. If this occurs, rehabilitation programs better tailored to LVAD patients should be designed.

Yanase et al. [44] reported that short term, such as 3-month rehabilitation program, could significantly increase post-HTx exercise capacity irrespective of age, gender, type of LVAD, and underlying disease. But, even in those patients, better several nutrition factors at exercise program admission were significantly associated with peak VO2 at the end of the exercise program. Therefore, nutrition supplementation during LVAD support might be also essential to improve exercise capacity post-HTx as well as exercise training. However, there are no guidelines regarding the best way to cardiac exercise prescription, especially for CF-LVAD patients. As a result, LVAD patients currently undergo rehabilitation protocols designed for other types of cardiovascular diseases or cardiac surgeries.

As patients receiving LVAD are deeply deconditioned due to advanced HF, it is recommended that patients with sarcopenia as well as frailty are admitted to an in-patient rehabilitation program soon after implanting LVAD. Alsara et al. [50] reviewed the literatures regarding cardiac rehabilitation in patients supported with LVAD and concluded that exercise training is safe and recommended early mobilization between 7 and 10 days post-LVAD and treadmill exercise training beginning at 21 days post-LVAD. However, there is very few information regarding the improvements derived from exercise training in LVAD patients.

Currently, pulsatile-flow LVADs (PF-LVADs) are seldom used as durable support in patients with end-stage HF, but they have a pneumatically/electrically driven ventricle operating in the complete fill/ and empty mode. Therefore, cardiac output during exercise will increase by an automatic increase in pump rate responding to an increase in left ventricular (LV) preload. PF-LVADs work independently from LV afterload and produce a maximal cardiac output of 10 liters/min with a pump rate of 120 beats/min [51]. On the other hand, the CF-LVAD has no inflow or outflow valves, unloads the ventricle in both systole and diastole, and operates at a fixed pump speed. The two types of CF-LVADs are axial and centrifugal. Pump flow changes according to the differential pressure between the inflow and outflow cannulas. The sensitivity of axial and centrifugal pumps to changes in preload is similar, whereas centrifugal pumps are more sensitive to afterload [52]. During exercise, pump flow increases in the CF-LVAD according to changes in LV preload and afterload. For example, RV failure decreases LV preload and high systemic pressure decreases LV afterload, resulting in reduced pump flow. Therefore, CF-LVAD cannot fully increase pump flow with exercise, whereas PF-LVAD can do so.

Haft et al. [53] reported the differences in the exercise hemodynamic responses between PF-LVAD and CF-LVAD. Peak VO2 as well as resting central venous pressure, mean arterial pressure, and pulmonary capillary wedge pressure were similar and pump flow increased peak VO2 in both groups. However, the increase in pump flow was approximately 20% greater in the PF-LVAD than in the CF-LVAD. Moreover, the significance of this finding is unclear because the pump flow through for the CF-LVAD is not directly measured but only estimated. Martina et al. [54] reported that patients supported with CF-LVAD showed a mean peak VO2 of 18 mL/kg/min (55% of predicted) and a mean total maximum cardiac output of 8.5 liters/min. From these studies, patients supported with CF-LVAD may have a similar peak VO2 independently of the type of CF-LVAD. Although maximum cardiac output increases with exercise in patients supported with CF-LVAD, it does not reach levels found in healthy individuals with normal cardiac function.

Many factors, such as underlying heart disease, native heart function, especially right ventricular function, both ventricular morphology, co-existing arrhythmia, type of LVAD, rehabilitation protocol, and nutrition intervention may influence the effect of cardiac rehabilitation on improvement in exercise capacity and recovery from sarcopenia. Therefore, individualized exercise prescriptions leading to optimal improvements in exercise capacity in patients supported with CF-LVAD are not well known and should be established in the field of LVAD therapy [47].

7.2 Nutrition

There is no doubt that malnutrition is involved in the pathogenesis of sarcopenia, and that it contributes to the poor muscle function observed in patients with end-stage HF, particularly in frail elderly patients. In general, the proposition of nutritional interventions should be based on the delivery of an adequate energy supply and on the supplementation of specific nutrients as an effective treatment in preventing and/or reversing sarcopenia in patients with advanced HF. However, there are very few literatures regarding the recovery from sarcopenia by nutrition interventions particularly in patients supported by LVAD.

8. Conclusion

Sarcopenia as well as frailty is a strong negative predictor on outcome after LVAD implantation and HTx. Assessment of skeletal muscle function such as HGS and gait speed, and measurement of skeletal muscle mass and CER index prior to surgery are useful tools to predict patient's outcome after LVAD implantation and HTx. Therefore, therapeutic strategies to reverse sarcopenia prior to surgery and after LVAD implantation are important to improve their outcomes. However, many factors, such as the indication, surgical method, postoperative therapies, and possible adverse events, might affect the efficacy of cardiac rehabilitation and nutrition supplementation on quality of life as well as survival differently in HTx and LVAD patients. Therefore, individualized exercise prescriptions and nutrition interventions leading to the reversal of sarcopenia as well as frailty in patients undergoing and supported with CF-LVAD should be established in the near future.

Author details

Norihide Fukushima
Department of Transplant Medicine, National Cerebral and Cardiovascular Center, Suita, Osaka

*Address all correspondence to: nori@ncvc.go.jp

IntechOpen

References

[1] Writing Group Members, Mozaffarian D, Benjamin EJ, Go AS, Arnett DK, Blaha MJ, et al. Executive summary: Heart disease and stroke statistics —2016 update: A report from the American Heart Association. Circulation. 2016;**133**:447-454

[2] Seferović PM. Introduction to the special issue entitled 'Heart failure management of the elderly patient: Focus on frailty, sarcopenia, cachexia, and dementia'. European Heart Journal Supplements: Journal of the European Society of Cardiology. 2019;**21**:L1-L3

[3] Saitoh M, Dos Santos MR, Ebner N, Emami A, Konishi M, Ishida J, et al. Nutritional status and its effects on muscle wasting in patients with chronic heart failure: Insights from studies investigating co-morbidities aggravating heart failure. Wiener Klinische Wochenschrift. 2016;**128**:1-8

[4] Sandek A, Doehner W, Anker SD, Von Haehling S. Nutrition in heart failure: An update. Current Opinion in Clinical Nutrition and Metabolic Care. 2009;**12**:384-391

[5] Cruz-Jentoft AJ, Landi F, Schneider SM, Zúñiga C, Arai H, Boirie Y, et al. Prevalence of and interventions for sarcopenia in ageing adults: A systematic review. Report of the International Sarcopenia Initiative (EWGSOP and IWGS). Age and Ageing. 2014;**43**:748-775

[6] Fonseca G, Dos Santos MR, de Souza FR, Takayama L, Rodrigues Pereira RM, Negrao CE, et al. Discriminating sarcopenia in overweight/obese male patients with heart failure: The influence of body mass index. ESC Heart Failure. 2020;7:84-91

[7] Bekfani T, Pellicori P, Morris DA, Ebner N, Valentova M, Steinbeck L,

et al. Sarcopenia in patients with heart failure with preserved ejection fraction: Impact on muscle strength, exercise capacity and quality of life. International Journal of Cardiology. 2016;**222**:41-46

[8] Curcio F, Testa G, Liguori I, Papillo M, Abete P. Sarcopenia and heart failure. Nutrients. 2020;**12**:211

[9] Mauro Z, Andrea R, Francesca C, Clara B, Gloria M, Francesco F. Sarcopenia, cachexia and congestive heart failure in the elderly. Endocr Metab Immune Disord - Drug Targets (Formerly Current Dru). 2013;**13**:58-67

[10] Fulster S, Tacke M, Sandek A, Ebner N, Tschope C, Doehner W, et al. Muscle wasting in patients with chronic heart failure: Results from the studies investigating co-morbidities aggravating heart failure (SICA-HF). European Heart Journal. 2013;**34**(7):512-519. DOI: 10.1093/eurheartj/ehs381

[11] Hajahmadi M, Shemshadi S, Khalilipur E, Amin A, Taghavi S, Maleki M, et al. Muscle wasting in young patients with dilated cardiomyopathy. Journal of Cachexia, Sarcopenia and Muscle. 2017;**8**(4): 542-548. DOI: 10.1002/jcsm.12193

[12] Anker SD, Chua TP, Ponikowski P, Harrington D, Swan JW, Kox WJ, et al. Hormonal changes and catabolic/ anabolic imbalance in chronic heart failure and their importance for cardiac cachexia. Circulation. 1997;**96**:526-534

[13] Osterziel KJ, Strohm O, Schuler J, Friedrich M, Hanlein D, Willenbrock R, et al. Randomised, double-blind, placebo-controlled trial of human recombinant growth hormone in patients with chronic heart failure due to dilated cardiomyopathy. Lancet. 1998;**351**(9111):1233-1237

[14] Hambrecht R, Schulze PC, Gielen S, Linke A, Mobius-Winkler S, Erbs S, et al. Effects of exercise training on insulin-like growth factor-I expression in the skeletal muscle of non-cachectic patients with chronic heart failure. European Journal of Cardiovascular Prevention and Rehabilitation. 2005;**12**(4):401-406

[15] Miller LW, Pagani FD, Russell SD, John R, Boyle AJ, Aaronson KD, et al. Use of a continuous-flow device in patients awaiting heart transplantation. The New England Journal of Medicine. 2007;**357**(9):885-896

[16] Park SJ, Milano CA, Tatooles AJ, Rogers JG, Adamson RM, Steidley DE, et al. Outcomes in advanced heart failure patients with left ventricular assist devices for destination therapy. Circulation. Heart Failure. 2012;**5**(2):241-248

[17] Khan RS, Kato TS, Chokshi A, Chew M, Yu S, Wu C, et al. Adipose tissue inflammation and adiponectin resistance in patients with advanced heart failure: Correction after ventricular assist device implantation. Circulation. Heart Failure. 2012;**5**(3):340-348

[18] Mancini D, Goldsmith R, Levin H, Beniaminovitz A, Rose E, Catanese K, et al. Comparison of exercise performance in patients with chronic severe heart failure versus left ventricular assist devices. Circulation. 1998;**98**(12):1178-1183

[19] Estep JD, Starling RC, Horstmanshof DA, Milano CA, Selzman CH, Shah KB, et al. Risk assessment and comparative effectiveness of left ventricular assist device and medical management in ambulatory heart failure patients: Results from the ROADMAP study. Journal of the American College of Cardiology. 2015;**66**:1747-1761

[20] Cruz-Jentoft AJ, Baeyens JP, Bauer JM. et al; European Working Group on Sarcopenia in Older People. Sarcopenia: European consensus on definition and diagnosis: Report of the European Working Group on Sarcopenia in Older People. Age and Ageing. 2010;**39**(4):412-423

[21] Chung CJ, Wu C, Jones M, Kato TS, Dam TT, Givens RC, et al. Reduced handgrip strength as a marker of frailty predicts clinical outcomes in patients with heart failure undergoing ventricular assist device placement. Journal of Cardiac Failure. 2014;**20**:310e315

[22] Khawaja T, Chokshi A, Ji R, Kato TS, Xu K, Zizola C, et al. Ventricular assist device implantation improves skeletal muscle function, oxidative capacity, and growth hormone/insulin-like growth factor-1 axis signaling in patients with advanced heart failure. Journal of Cachexia, Sarcopenia and Muscle. 2014;**5**:297-305

[23] Lee JS, He K, Harbaugh CM, Schaubel DE, Sonnenday CJ, Wang SC, et al. Frailty, core muscle size, and mortality in patients undergoing open abdominal aortic aneurysm repair. Journal of Vascular Surgery. 2011;**53**:912e917

[24] Englesbe MJ, Patel SP, He K, Lynch RJ, Schaubel DE, Harbaugh C, et al. Sarcopenia and mortality after liver transplantation. Journal of the American College of Surgeons. 2010;**211**:271e278

[25] Sheetz KH, Zhao L, Holcombe SA, Wang SC, Reddy RM, Lin J, et al. Decreased core muscle size is associated with worse patient survival following esophagectomy for cancer. Diseases of the Esophagus. 2013;**26**:716e722

[26] Peng P, Hyder O, Firoozmand A, Kneuertz P, Schulick RD, Huang D, et al. Impact of sarcopenia on outcomes

following resection of pancreatic adenocarcinoma. Journal of Gastrointestinal Surgery. 2012;**16**:1478e1486

[27] Buess D, Kressig RW. Sarcopenia: Definition, diagnostics and therapy. Praxis. 2013;**102**:1167-1170

[28] Drexler H, Riede U, Munzel T, Konig H, Funke E, Just H. Alterations of skeletal muscle in chronic heart failure. Circulation. 1992;**85**:1751-1759

[29] Bhanji RA, Carey EJ, Yang L, Watt KD. The long winding road to transplant: How sarcopenia and debility impact morbidity and mortality on the waitlist. Clinical Gastroenterology and Hepatology. 2017;**15**(10):1492-1497

[30] Kim EY, Kim YS, Park I, Ahn HK, Cho EK, Jeong YM, et al. Evaluation of sarcopenia in small-cell lung cancer patients by routine chest CT. Support Care Cancer. 2016;**24**:4721-4726

[31] Kim YS, Kim EY, Kang SM, Ahn HK, Kim HS. Single cross-sectional area of pectoralis muscle by computed tomography: Correlation with bioelectrical impedance based skeletal muscle mass in healthy subjects. Clinical Physiology and Functional Imaging. 2017;**37**:507-511

[32] Teigen LM, John R, Kuchnia AJ, Nagel EM, Earthman CP, Kealhofer J, et al. Preoperative pectoralis muscle quantity and attenuation by computed tomography are novel and powerful predictors of mortality after left ventricular assist device implantation. Circulation. Heart Failure. 2017;**10**:e004069

[33] Beddhu S, Pappas LM, et al. Effects of body size and body composition on survival in hemodialysis patients. Journal of the American Society of Nephrology. 2003;**14**:2366-2372

[34] ter Maaten JM, Damman K, et al. Creatinine excretion rate, a marker of

muscle mass, is related to clinical outcome in patients with chronic systolic heart failure. Clinical Research in Cardiology. 2014;**103**:976-983

[35] Poortmans JR, Boisseau N, et al. Estimation of total-body skeletal muscle mass in children and adolescents. Medicine and Science in Sports and Exercise. 2005;**37**:316-322

[36] Iwasaki K, Seguchi O, Murata S, et al. Effect of the creatinine excretion rate index, a marker of sarcopenia, on prediction of intracranial hemorrhage in patients with advanced heart failure and a continuous-flow left ventricular assist device. Circulation Journal. 2020;**84**(6):949-957

[37] Heberton GA, Nassif M, Bierhals A, Novak A, LaRue SJ, Lima B, et al. Usefulness of psoas muscle area determined by computed tomography to predict mortality or prolonged length of hospital stay in patients undergoing left ventricular assist device implantation. The American Journal of Cardiology. 2016;**118**:1363e1367

[38] Hydren JR, Corwell WK, Richardson RS, Drako SD. Exercise capacity in mechanically supported advanced heart failure patients: It is all about the beat. ASAIO Journal. 2020;**66**(4):339-342. DOI: 10.1097/MAT.0000000000001164

[39] Cogswell R, Trachtenberg B, Murray T, Schultz J, Teigen L, Allen T, et al. A novel model incorporating pectoralis muscle measures to predict mortality after ventricular assist device implantation. Journal of Cardiac Failure. 2020;**26**:308-315

[40] Tsuji M, Amiya E, Hatano M, et al. Abdominal skeletal muscle mass as a predictor of mortality in Japanese patients undergoing left ventricular assist device implantation. ESC Heart Fail 2019;**6**(3):526-535.

[41] Cogswell R, Estep JD, AraujoGutierrez R, Masotti M, Majaraj V, Teigen L, et al. Heart failure severity stratification beyond INTERMACS profiles: A step toward optimal left ventricular assist device timing. ASAIO Journal. 2021;**67**(5):554-560

[42] Cooper LB, Lu D, Mentz RJ, et al. Cardiac transplantation for older patients: Characteristics and outcomes in the septuagenarian population. The Journal of Heart and Lung Transplantation. 2016;**35**:362-369

[43] Flint KM, Matlock DD, Lindenfeld J, et al. Frailty and the selection of patients for destination therapy left ventricular assist device. Circulation. Heart Failure. 2012;**5**(2):286-293

[44] Yanase M, Seguchi O, Nakanishi M, et al. The role of three-month program of rehabilitative exercise after heart transplantation: The effects of the recipient's and donor's risk. International Journal of Physical Medicine & Rehabilitation. 2019;**6**:6. DOI: 10.4172/2329-9096.1000503

[45] Jha SR, Hannu MK, Newton PJ, et al. Reversibility of frailty after bridge-to-transplant ventricular assist device implantation or heart transplantation. Transplantation direct. 2017;**3**(7):e167

[46] Macdonald P. Frailty of the Heart Recipient. Transplantation. 2021 Feb 11. doi: 10.1097/TP.0000000000003692. Online ahead of print.

[47] Maurer MS, Horn E, Reyentovich A, et al. Can a left ventricular assist device in individuals with advanced systolic heart failure improve or reverse frailty? Journal of the American Geriatrics Society. 2017;**65**(11):2383-2390

[48] Fernandes L, Oliveira IM, Fernandes PF, de Souza Neto JD, Farias M, Freitas NA, et al. Impact of heart transplantation on the recovery of peripheral and respiratory muscle mass and strength in patients with chronic heart failure. Transplantation direct. 2018;**4**(11):e395. DOI: 10.1097/TXD.0000000000000837

[49] Schaufelberger M, Eriksson BO, Lönn L, et al. Skeletal muscle characteristics, muscle strength and thigh muscle area in patients before and after cardiac transplantation. European Journal of Heart Failure. 2001;**3**:59-67

[50] Alsara O, Perez-Terzic C, Squires RW, et al. Is exercise training safe and beneficial in patients receiving left ventricular assist device therapy? Journal of Cardiopulmonary Rehabilitation and Prevention. 2014;**34**:233-240

[51] Hunt SA, Frazier OH. Mechanical circulatory support and cardiac transplantation. Circulation. 1998;**97**:2079-2090

[52] Moazami N, Fukamachi K, Kobayashi M, et al. Axial and centrifugal continuous-flow rotary pumps: A translation from pump mechanics to clinical practice. The Journal of Heart and Lung Transplantation. 2013;**32**:1-11

[53] Haft J, Armstrong W, Dyke DB, et al. Hemodynamic and exercise performance with pulsatile and continuous-flow left ventricular assist devices. Circulation. 2007;**116**:I8-I15

[54] Martina J, de Jonge N, Rutten M, et al. Exercise hemodynamics during extended continuous flow left ventricular assist device support: The response of systemic cardiovascular parameters and pump performance. Artificial Organs. 2013;**37**:754-762

Management of Sarcopenic Patients

Chapter 4

Sarcopenia: Technological Advances in Measurement and Rehabilitation

Letizia Lorusso, Luigi Esposito, Daniele Sancarlo and Grazia D'Onofrio

Abstract

Sarcopenia is an important recently defined disease affecting people aged ≥ 65 years all over the world. Improving the assessment of loss of muscle mass is becoming mandatory. In this regard, various new technologies have been advanced. Although the gold standard is represented by magnetic resonance imaging (MRI) or magnetic resonance spectroscopy (MRS), computed tomography (CT) or dual-energy X-ray absorptiometry (DXA), followed by biological impedance analysis (BIA) compared with DXA, there are numerous correlations between sarcopenia and health domain of everyday life that must be investigated and addressed, trying to obtain the best possible outcome in the older population. In this review, we focused on all types of new technologies assessing loss of muscle mass, frailty, independence, walking, capacity to get dressed, and loss of balance or sleepiness in older people and that could improve the diagnosis of sarcopenia or the rehabilitation of sarcopenic patients to prevent possible accidents. Different technologies have been proposed to investigate the factors promoting the loss of muscle mass and weakness. Despite the standard EWGSOP 2019 guidelines defining a specific methodology for the diagnosis of sarcopenia, not all domains and devices were included, and new frontiers of prevention have been explored.

Keywords: new technologies, sarcopenia, measurement, rehabilitation, device

1. Introduction

Sarcopenia was defined by the International Classification of Diseases, Tenth Revision, Clinical Modification (ICD-10-CM) and recognized as a disease in 2016 [1–3]. In 2019, the European Working Group on Sarcopenia in Older People (EWGSOP) published important recommendations for the diagnosis of Sarcopenia for Caucasian People [4]. These recommendations are currently used as guidelines for the assessment of sarcopenia.

The first guidelines for the diagnosis of sarcopenia were written on the occasion of the first EWGSOP Congress in 2010 [5]. They also included some criteria for the diagnosis of *pre-sarcopenia* (loss of muscle mass and its variability).

The functional and anatomical areas to investigate for diagnosis, defined in both the first and second EWGSOP Congress [4], are muscle strength (hereinafter referred to as MS); muscle quality (hereinafter referred to as MQ), and physical performance (hereinafter referred to as PP). Nowadays, in accordance with the second EWGSOP guidelines, MS is evaluated through the assessment of grip strength (subsequently referred to as handgrip strength or HGS). The dynamometer is an inexpensive and efficient tool, but it investigates only the strength exerted by the upper limbs and has several limitations [6]. The recommended tests for MQ are magnetic resonance imaging (MRI) or magnetic resonance spectroscopy (MRS); computed tomography (CT); dual-energy X-ray absorptiometry (DXA) [4], including the alternative use of the biological impedance analysis (BIA) [7]. Regarding PP, the suggested gold standards are the short physical performance battery (SPPB) combined with the time-up and go test (TUG), or, as an alternative, the gait speed test (GS) [4].

However, the problem is that DXA, MRI, and BIA are not always available in hospitals and at the surgeries of general practitioners, and are fairly expensive.

Therefore, the aim of this review is to suggest some new and less expensive tools and technologies that may substitute the three tests mentioned above and that are able to maintain a reliable level of diagnostic accuracy. Moreover, we would like to extend the MS parameters not only to the upper limbs but also to the lower limbs and to the assessment of balance and spatial coordination. The use of these accurate and cheaper tools would favor the diagnosis of sarcopenia and, consequently, the prevention of loss of muscle mass, in a higher number of patients. Alternative tools for the evaluation of MS and PP as well as some rehabilitation tools for the prevention of bad outcomes in pre-sarcopenic and sarcopenic patients will also be proposed.

2. Methodology

This is a review of five randomized control trials (RCT), three cohort studies (CS), 13 cross-sectional studies (CSS), two systematic reviews (SR), two systematic reviews & meta-analyses (SR&M), one quasi-experimental study (Q-ES), one design and validation study (DVS), one exploratory study (ES), four randomized control studies (RCS), and four articles on new integrated technologies, some of which not yet tested on humans. The research was carried out between April 2021 and July 2021. The following libraries were searched: PubMed, Cochrane Library, Google Scholar, and Scopus.

A total of 6069 records were obtained. Of these, 5931 were discarded: 1833 were duplicates and 4098 were eliminated because of the type of population or because they focused on populations affected by cancer, or having post-operative outcomes or head and neck cancer with post-surgical outcomes affecting the tongue, or because they were studies based the use of ultrasound, MRI, CT, and DXA. Also, we excluded papers dealing with the rehabilitation of sarcopenia after a hip fracture or other similar events.

The eligibility criteria were: (1) community-dwelling older adults; (2) older adult volunteers: out-patient or hospitalized patients; (3) frail subjects according to the frailty criteria defined by Fried et al. [8]. About age, some of the studies focused on patients aged ≥50 years (middle-aged), others on patients aged ≥65 years (older), and others on patients aged 19 to an older age. Studies that did not include older adults were excluded.

Works referring to the Asian Working Group for Sarcopenia guidelines were also excluded.

Moreover, of the remaining 138 articles, 102 were discarded because they were duplicates or because they were not pertinent to the aim of the research.

The studies analyzed for this review were 36: 32 dealing with tested technologies whose results were compared with the parameters established in the EWGSOP guidelines, and four studies presenting new and not tested technologies.

The article search was carried out by using the following word strings and the PubMed's Boolean operators: *"phase angle and sarcopenia"*; *"rehabilitation and* sarcopenia"; "sarcopenia and measurement"; "actigraphy and sarcopenia"; "jumping mechanography"; "sarcopenia and wearable devices"; "sarcopenia robotic measurements". The search was restricted to the 2015–2021 period, including extremes.

To assess the quality of the paper, the Newcastle-Ottawa quality assessment scale was used [9].

3. Results

3.1 Diagnosis and rehabilitation of sarcopenia

3.1.1 Assessment of sarcopenia

3.1.1.1 Accelerometer and actigraph technology in wearable inertial sensors

Nowadays, wearable inertial sensors have the potential to assess MQ and PP (**Table 1**) [15].

In 2018, the American Academy of Sleep Medicine recommended using the actigraphy test for the diagnosis of sleep disorders [16]. Subsequently, on the basis of the ascertained association between frailty domains and functional limitations [8, 12, 17], Pana et al. investigated the relationship between sleep quality and MS among community-dwelling middle-aged and older adults [12]. The existence of a correlation between sleep disorders and sarcopenia can be expected but, until now, research in this field has been fragmented and no studies have been carried out investigating a possible direct correlation between sleep disorders and sarcopenia. For example, a study [18] has been published on the correlation between peak oxygen consumption and muscle loss. Physiological data were obtained through a feature of the actigraphy test called Actihear [19] which, however, focused on muscular functionality and not on sleep quality.

Accelerometer has been proposed in wearable devices to assess different parameters of physical activity following the "The Physical Activity Guidelines for Americans" (PAG, 2nd edition) [13], as shown in **Table 1**. However, in two studies in which the accelerometry was used, the accelerometry threshold did not prove to be indicative [10, 11]. Viecelli et al. [20] used a smartphone built-in accelerometer to obtain scientific mechano-biological descriptors of resistance exercise training. They aimed to test whether accelerometer data obtained from standard smartphone placed on the weight stack of resistance exercise machines can be used to extract single repetition, contraction-phase specific and total time-under-tension (TUT) [20]. Total time-under-tension is an important mechano-biological descriptor of resistance exercise as it was shown that it is highly positive correlated ($R2 = 0.99$) with the phosphorylation c-Jun N-terminal kinase (JNK) [21]. Activated JNK phosphorylates the transcription factor SMAD2, leading to the inhibition of myostatin [22], a potent negative regulator of muscle mass [23, 24]. The JNK/SMAD signaling axis is activated by resistance exercise and hence the molecular switch JNK stimulates muscle fiber growth, resulting in increased muscle mass [22] being a direct countermeasure of the muscle loss seen in sarcopenia.

Burd et al. [25] examined the influence of muscle time-under-tension on myofibrillar protein synthesis. Eight young men were allocated into two groups. One group performed three sets of unilateral knee extension at 30% of 1-repetition maximum involving concentric and eccentric muscle actions that were 6 s in duration to failure. The control group performed a work-matched bout that comprised concentric and eccentric actions that were 1 s in duration. As work was matched, the groups significantly differed in time-under-tension ($P < 0.001$) whereby the slow group had a time-under-tension of

Author, year, country	Study design	Sample Mean Age ± SD	Technologies employed	Data collected/ performed measurement	Session modality
Foong et al., 2016; Australia [10]	CSS	636 community-dwelling OA: 66 ± 7 years	ACC technology to assess PA	AMM S-ACC CF	Monitoring of PA at baseline, and 2.7 years, 5 years later, and last follow-up; between March 2002 and September 2004, ending on 2014
Rejeski et al., 2017; USA [11]	CSS	1.528 OA: HE (*N* = 771): 79.07 ± 5.23 and PA (*N* = 757): 78.74 ± 5.21	GT3X+ accelerometer: CPM to assess MVPA.	HE (*N* = 771) PA (*N* = 757) divided for: • Health-related variables education • SPPB • EFs	Data examined at baseline, and 6-, 12-, and 24-months of follow-up
Pana et al., 2021; Greece [12]	SR	92.363 OA ≥65 years and middle-aged adults ≥ 40 years	ASD	HGS SAss	Research from March 2020 to May 2020
Zytnick et al., 2021; USA [13]	R-CSS	1.317 healthy adults aged ≥60 years	WAM	Data collected from the fall wave of the 2015 styles database: FallStyles: PA and walking	Data monitoring, data activity carried out for more than 12 months
Kim et al., 2021; Korea [14]	CS	20 older women aged ≥65 years: 10 sarcopenic women with: 69.6 ± 3.0 and 10 normal women with: 71.1 ± 2.0	IS	GS, HGS, and walking to analyze raw data, it will be applied DL methods	Acquiring spatial-temporal parameters used in clinical practice and descriptive statistical parameters for all seven gait phases

CSS, cross-sectional studies; CS, cohort studies; SR, systematic review; R-CSS, retrospective-cross-sectional studies; OA; older adults; PA, physical activity; CPM, counts per minute; MVPA, moderate to vigorous PA; HE, health education; DH, digital handgrip; DYN, dynamometer; ACC, accelerometer; ASD, actigraphy sleep diary; WAM, wearable activity monitor; IS, inertial sensors; AMM, anthropometrics muscle mass; S-ACC, strength accelerometer; CF, cognitive function; SPPB, short physical performance battery; TUG, time-up and go test; EFs, executive functions; MS, maximal strength; RFD, rate of force development; SA, strength asymmetry; BS, bilateral strength; FSFT-ST, force steadiness fatigability task-specific tremor; HGS, hand grip strength; GS, gait speed; SAss, sleep assessment; DL, deep learning.

Table 1.
General overview of the paper focused on the accelerometer in wearable devices and the actual use of actigraphy to assess sarcopenia in primary prevention.

407 ± 23 s and the control group a time-under-tension 50 ± 3, respectively. Myofibrillar protein synthetic rate was higher in the slow condition versus the control condition after 24–30 h recovery (P < 0.001). Therefore, a longer time-under-tension increased myofibrillar protein synthesis longer and to a greater extent than under the control condition.

As evident, time-under-tension is not only an important mechano-biological descriptor of resistance exercise but also of high clinical relevance.

Lastly, a very recent article [14] aimed at identifying and elaborating parameters from gait signals produced by the sensors in order to develop a screening and classification method for sarcopenia. In the study were used specific parameters that they interpreted through an artificial intelligence (AI) model called SHAP (*Shapley Additive Explanations*). The input that applied the SHAP to the descriptive statistical parameters

Author, year, country	Study design	Sample Mean Age ± SD	Technologies employed	Data collected/ performed measurement	Session modality
Swiecicka et al., 2019; UK [17]	RCT	86 older men aged 74 ± 5.	EMG (DS7AH; Digitimer, Welwyn Garden City, UK); AAE (Dermatrode, Farmadomo, The Netherlands); S2S (v.8.1; Cambridge Electronic Designs).	L&NBRM determined relationship between FP and FI with CMAP and MUP sizes before and after adjustments for age and BMI.	The femoral nerve was stimulated maximally and the resulting CMAP measured over the vastus lateralis. MUP size assessed in voluntary contractions using (iEMG).
Habenicht et al., 2020; Vienna [26]	CSS	86 VHP between 18 and 90 years of age.	BED and EMG (DAVID®, Helsinki, Finland); EMG (Model Trigno, DelSys®, Boston, MA, USA) and TXACC-SI.	Anthropometric measurements, IPAQ, warm-up and MVC, HGS, and EMG.	Measurement obtained during training session: first session at baseline, second session 2 days after, and third session 6 weeks later.
Marshall et al., 2020 [27]	CSS	15 HY: 25 ± 3 years; and 15 OA: 70 ± 5 years.	BIA (mBCA 525, SECA, Hamburg, Germany); EMG (Mbody, Myontec Ltd., Kuopio, Finland).	Indices of QM EMG activity in response to different modes of RET and ADL.	In 4 days, participants completed a MVC of the KE, followed by a 15mWT, SCT (i.e., ADL) and BW-RET and MN-RET or EB-RET.
Gennaro et al., 2020; Switzerland [28]	ES	198 community-dwelling volunteers: 73 ± 6 years.	EMG: FREEEMG 1000, BTS Bioengineering, Milan, Italy; EEG: eego sport, ANT Neuro, Enschede, The Netherlands.	EEG and EMG samples in sarcopenic participants.	Acquired during walking, then processed.
Hu et al., 2021; Taiwan [29]	CSS	Five risk-sarcopenia (age: 66.20 ± 4.44), five healthy (age: 69.00 ± 2.35), and 20 young (age: 21.33 ± 1.15).	EMG (EMGworks® 4.0 Acquisition software, Delsys Inc., Boston, MA, USA).	EMG parameters as: MN_{RT}, MFR_{RT}, y-intercept, FRU, and mean MFR extracted to analyze MFD. HGS, GS, PASE, and IPAQ.	Not defined.

RCT, randomized control trials; CSS, cross-sectional studies; ES, exploratory study; VHP, voluntary health people; HY, healthy young; OA, older adults; BIA, biological impedance analysis; HGS, hand grip strength; EMG, electromyography; EEG, electroencephalogram; L&NBRM, logistic & negative binomial regression models; BED, back extension dynamometer; RET, resistance exercise training; KE, knee extension; SCT, stair climbing task; MVC, maximal voluntary contraction; 15mWT, 15 minutes walking task; TXACC-SI, triaxial accelerometer-sensor integrated; QM, quadriceps muscle; BW-RET, lower-limb RET through body-weight squats; MN-RET, seated knee extensions on machine; AAE, adhesive anode electrode; EB-RET, seated knee extensions via elastic bands; S2S, Spike2 Software; FP, frailty phenotype; FI, frailty index; CMAP, compound muscle action potential; MUP, motor unit potential; MN_{RT}, motor unit number-recruitment threshold; MFR_{RT}, motor unit firing rate-recruitment threshold; FRU, firing rate per unit force; MFR, motor unit firing rate; MFD, muscle fiber discrimination; PASE, physical activity of senior elder; IPAQ, International Physical Activity Questionnaire.

Table 2.
General overview of the paper focused on new tools for the assessment of sarcopenia with electromyography (EMG).

yielded the best performance; showing that the signal of the inertial sensor contained abundant information on gait parameters. However, the deep learning did not extract effective features from inertial signals; further data and greater cohorts, respectively, with additional clinical evaluations should be collected and studied [14].

3.1.1.2 Electromyography

In **Table 2**, an interesting new technology capable of evaluating variations in muscle activity is shown: the EMG.

It was demonstrated [17] that some electrophysiological sarcopenic variables were associated with the frailty phenotype [8, 17], but frailty in older men was associated with lower CMAP and MUP, which however were not related to age and BMI.

On the basis of the data obtained by Habenicht et al. [26] in their study on back extension, a diagnostic algorithm for assessing the first signs of muscle weakness

Author, year, country	Study design	Sample Mean Age ± SD	Technologies employed	Data collected/ performed measurement	Session modality
Dietzel et al., 2015; Germany [32]	CSS	Total of 293 C-D women (146) and men (147): aged 60–85 years.	Leonardo Mechanograph® (Novotec Medical, Pforzheim, Germany); plateDXA.	DXA data, ADL, JM, EFI, HF, CRT$_V$. MF: muscle power per 2LJP$_{rel}$ and the CRT$_{Prel}$ on a force.	30 subjects in each 5-year.
Siglinsky et al., 2015, Madison (USA) [33]	CS	USA OA (213 women/119 men), mean: 65.4 ± 17.4 years.	DXA, Leonardo Mechanograph®	BMI, ALM/Ht2, HGS, GS, CRT, JH, JRP, Vel. (m/s) APT.	Randomly.
Hannam et al., 2017; Bristol, UK [34]	CSS	463 C-D of which: 300 76.4 ± 2.6, and 163 with 77.7 ± 3.6 years.	Jumping Mechanography (Leonardo Mechanograph).	JM, SPPB, HGS.	Re-recruited participants from an earlier population-based cohort study, during 2015 for 1 years.
Minett et al., 2020; Germany [35]	RCT	94 OA: 46 users to the WALK: mean 75.8 years and 48 to the W + EX: mean 77.1 years.	DXA and JM.	F&C, weekly meetings, DI&EH, BIA, MD, M-CSA, IMAT, MF, and MM, JM.	3-month exercise intervention, measured performed at baseline and at the third month. 09-12/2016.
Alvero-Cruz et al., 2021; Málaga, Spain [36]	CSS	256 MATH of these, 240 ATH aged between 35 and 91 years; mean 58 ± 12 years.	BIA, JM.	Anthropometric, BIA, JM.	Between 4th and 15th September 2018, during the 23rd-WMAC held in Málaga; 40–60 minutes for athlete.

CSS, cross-sectional studies; CS, cohort studies; RCT, randomized control trials; OA, older adult; C-D, community-dwelling; JM, jumping mechanography; BIA, biological impedance analysis; DXA, dual-energy X-ray absorptiometry; BMI, body mass index; EFI, Esslinger fitness index; HF, history falls; MF, muscle function; 2LJP$_{rel}$, maximum 2 leg jump power per kg body mass; CRTP$_{rel}$, maximum chair rise test power per kg body mass; CRT $_V$, the max velocity of the CRT; HGS, hand-grip strength; GS, gait speed; SPPB, short physical performance battery; JRP, jumping relative power; APT, acceptability; W or WALK, walking; EX, exercises; F&C, feasibility & compliance; DI&EH, dietary intakes & eating habits; MD, muscle density; M-CSA, muscle cross-sectional area; IMAT, intramuscular adipose tissue; MM, mobility measures; MATH, masters athletes; ATH, athletes; 23RD-WMAC, 23rd-World Masters Athletics Championships.

Table 3.
General overview of papers based on jumping mechanography.

related to back extension may be developed [26]. Subsequently, Gennaro et al. [28], in their ES, defined "*corticomuscular coherence*" (CMC), obtained during locomotion by simultaneously measuring EEG and EMG, and suggested it as a new feature for the diagnosis of sarcopenia [28], reporting that it has a high sensitivity and specificity.

Marshall et al. [27] compared BW-RET with MN-RET and EB-RET in a group of healthy younger adults and a group of older adults: BW-RET proved less effective than MN-RET and EB-RET. The EMG parameters were defined by studying a population composed of young adults, healthy and at-risk older adults [29] (as shown in **Table 2**). In the article, they concluded that it was not clear if EMG difference correlates with MS loss or mere loss of muscle mass [29].

3.1.1.3 Jumping mechanography

The association between the jumping mechanography (JM) and sarcopenia starts with Buehring et al. [30, 31], who gave "operational definitions of the variables available through muscle mechanography" with the aim to propose muscle mechanography as a tool for what we defined as MQ parameter [31], supporting the reproducibility of JM in older people [30, 32].

To assess muscle function and, at the same time, the MQ and PP parameters, JM can be considered an interesting new tool. It was first described by Dietzel et al., Siglinsky et al., Hannam et al., and Gangnon et al. [30, 32–34]; in all of these studies, JM was performed by Leonardo Mechanograph® (**Table 3**). JM measures the peak of muscle power by a vertical jump, as this practice is considered safe and useful to assess not only MQ and PP parameters but also different geriatric outcomes clearly important in primary prevention.

In all previous studies, participants were tested in accordance with the first EWGSOP guidelines [32, 33] and showed a better correlation between ADL and JM performance. Such correlation gives useful indications for the prevention of falls and fractures. In another work [34], the feasibility and acceptability of JM were evaluated: JM was considered comfortable and the comfort was related to one's own JM performance.

Also, in the work by Alvero-Cruz et al. [36], sarcopenia was diagnosed according to the first EWGSOP guidelines. They did not use JM but studied highly trained track and field athletes to explain the age-related decline in vertical jumping performance, obtaining data from the Redcap, Leonardo, and BIA data merging [36].

Of interest, in 2020 a complete and well-designed RCT was carried out [35]. It consisted of an intervention program based on physical exercises to evaluate outcomes in anthropometrics, body composition, muscle function, mobility measures, JM, and dietary habits. It showed that the program could be feasible in a population of older adults and that JM detected differences in MS and MQ using the chair-rise test rather than the TUG test [35].

All the above-mentioned studies were carried out on the basis of the first EWGSOP guidelines. However, it is now necessary to perform studies comparing results with the second EWGSOP guidelines. Wiegmann et al. defined a diagnostic algorithm on the basis of the 2nd EWGSOP guidelines [37].

3.1.1.4 Sarcopenia and BIA's phase angle

The BIA's phase angle (PhA) was mentioned, not for the first time, in a work by Heymsfield et al. [7]. Biological impedance analysis (BIA) was considered a useful tool for sarcopenic patients who were unable to perform a handgrip test or to walk [4, 38, 39]. Nowadays, BIA is used to confirm the diagnosis of sarcopenia (**Table 4**).

Author, year, country	Study design	Sample Mean Age ± SD	Technologies employed	Data collected/ performed measurement	Session modality
Pessoa et al., 2019; Brazil [40]	CSS	94 physically active older women: Tercile 1 (*n* = 31): 73.5 ± 7.6 Terciles 2 and 3 (*n* = 63): 69.6 ± 5.7	BIA (Biodynamics® 450, version 5.1).	BIA and PhA; 4-mWST, HGS, following 1st EWGSOP criteria.	Not specified.
Rosas-Carrasco et al., 2021; Mexico [41]	CS	498 Mexican older adults with over 50 years of age 71.1 ± 9.5.	BIA (SECAR model mBCA 514.), DXA and DYN.	BIA and PhA; HGS, DXA, CES, MMSE, MNA-SF.	Cohort of adults living in the community of two municipalities of Mexico City consisting of men and women over 50 years of age.

CSS, cross-sectional studies; CS, cohort studies; BIVA, bioelectrical impedance vector analysis; BIA, biological impedance analysis; DXA, dual-energy X-ray absorptiometry; 4-mWST, 4-m walking speed test; HGS, hand-grip strength; CES, center for epidemiologic studies, DS, depression scale (Mexican version); MMSE, mini-mental state examination; MNA-SF, mini nutritional assessment-short form; PhA, phase angle; NRS-2002, Nutritional Risk Screening 2002; DT, drawing test.

Table 4.
General overview of the relationship between the assessment of sarcopenia and BIA's phase angle.

Author, year, country	Study design	Sample Mean Age ± SD	Technologies employed	Data collected/ performed measurement	Session modality
Beveridge et al., 2018, Scotland, UK [42]	RCT	SC-D people >65 years, Study 1: 77.6 ± 6.2; for study 2, and data of study 1.	Magstim 200 system (Magstim Company Ltd., Whitland, UK).	6 MW, QMVC, SPPB, HGS and TwQ compared with population of Study 2.	Stimulation at baseline and 2 weeks along with 6 MW, QMVC, SPPB and HG.
Lera et al., 2020; Chile [43]	DVS	430 C-D people 60 years and older: 68.2 ± 4.9	Mobile devices (Android, IOS) and software HTSMayor.	EWGSOP parameters compared with software.	A comparison between clinical diagnosis and software diagnosis, with a median follow-up of 4.8 years.
Bachasson et al., 2021; France [44]	CSS	40 of which 20 HP: 8 women, aged 37 ± 9 years, and 12 men, age 35 ± 10 years; and 20 SP: 10 men, aged 63 ± 7 years and 10 women, aged 68 ± 10 years.	MRI using a 3 T Scanner (PrismaFit, Siemens, Healthineers, Erlangen, Germany), BIA (Z-Scan, Bioparhom, France).	Lean thigh muscle volume from MRI (IV_{MRI}) compared with lean thigh muscle volume from BIA (IV_{BIA}).	IV_{MRI} was computed, subsequently, multifrequency acquired. Values of the muscle electrical conductivity constant were computed using data from S_{BIA} and MRI.

CSS, cross-sectional study; RCT, random controlled trial; SC-D, sarcopenic community-dueling; C-D, community-dueling; DVS, design and validation study; HP, healthy participants; SP, sarcopenic participants; BIA, biological impedance analysis; MRI, magnetic resonance imaging; 6 MW, six minutes walking; QMVC, maximum voluntary quadriceps contraction; TwQ, maximum quadriceps twitch tension.

Table 5.
General overview of the paper focused on the assessment of sarcopenia: New tools and software.

According to a study carried out in Mexico [40] on active older women, there seems to be no correlation between PhA and sarcopenia parameters, but PhA seems to be associated, with a doubtful biological meaning, with speed walking [40] (or PP). In a recent paper [41], they analyzed sarcopenia on the basis of the parameters defined by the second EWGSOP guidelines, and physical frailty, according to the parameters defined by Fried et al. [8], both adjusted to the Mexican population.

Studies on more homogeneous populations may clarify the usefulness of BIA's PhA.

3.1.1.5 New technologies tested

Magstim 200 system: Magnetic nerve stimulation was tested on older sarcopenic people [42]. The study reports several limitations in the execution and screening of sarcopenic patients whose functions were not highly compromised. Despite this and the fact that it is an expensive technique, this methodology is still considered acceptable and feasible. More tests on sarcopenic patients with highly impaired functionality would be needed (**Table 5**).

Software HTSMavor: In South America, accessibility to DXA is very difficult. With the purpose to facilitate the assessment of sarcopenia, a screening algorithm for the diagnosis of sarcopenia, following the second EWGSOP guidelines, was developed. The results are very promising, but software accuracy for different populations should be implemented [43].

Bioelectrical impedance analysis to estimate the lean muscle volume: Serial bioelectrical impedance analysis (S_{BIA}) was compared with magnetic resonance imaging (MRI) [44]. As a strong agreement between IV_{BIA} and IV_{MRI} was found, a specific conductivity constant (σ) was computed in order to assess the reliability of S_{BIA} as a possible alternative to MRI. Despite the study limitations, the technique appears to be very promising.

3.1.2 Rehabilitation in sarcopenia

Sarcopenic patients are not usually followed in the daily routine, therefore it would be advisable to develop rehabilitation programs to keep the progression of the disease under control. Rehabilitation programs usually contain enhanced physical exercises and dietary increased amounts of protein intake [45]. In the absence of these rehabilitation programs, physicians give advice on physical exercises and dietary habits to patients. However, these recommendations are rarely observed by the patients [46].

In the following part of this manuscript, we talk about new proposals on rehabilitation. Such proposals include new or old technologies that could be used in planned therapies for pre-sarcopenic and sarcopenic patients.

3.1.2.1 Virtual reality and laser therapy

Thousands of articles on rehabilitation protocols that use virtual reality in different research fields have been produced [47, 48], but there are still few studies applying virtual reality to sarcopenia. The patients on whom the usability was tested were older patients with varied pathologies. The results were promising; therefore, it is hoped that it will be applicable to sarcopenic patients (**Table 6**).

In the work by Chen et al. [50], the virtual reality-based progressive resistance training was tested on patients residing in a nursing home, over a period of 12 weeks. The outcomes were different, but the training determined an improvement especially of the upper limb strength, in other words, MS and MQ but not PP. An increase of ASMM was present but was not statistically significant [50]. Further studies are required.

Author, year, country	Study design	Sample Mean Age ± SD	Technologies employed	Data collected/ performed measurement	Session modality
Toma et al., 2016; Brazil [49]	RCT-DB	38 elderly women: -CG = 15; 63.64 ± 2.11- TG = 17; mean: 63.31 ± 2.66- TLG = 16; mean: 64.07 ± 2.87.	An infrared AsGaAl laser (λ = 808 nm) (Photon Lase III; DMC® São Carlos, SP, Brazil).	6-MWT, SEMG, 1-RM, BS, IP.	STS was performed by TG and TLG groups for 8 consecutive weeks. Placebo or active LLLT for CG at the end of each STS.
Chen et al., 2020; Taiwan, China [50]	Q-ES	30 residents: 74.57.	VR-RHE; ORH; one constellation; LMS.	HGS, GS, BIA.	Measurements at baseline, and at 4, 8, and 12 weeks. Session took place twice per week, 30 minutes per session.
Tuena et al., 2021; Portugal [47]	SR	405 OA and YA and other specific disease patients.	VR: 3D simulator environment system.	SUS, other questionnaires, and physical impairments.	Variable

RTC-DB, randomized control trial-double blinded; Q-ES, quasi-experimental study; SR, systematic review; VR-RHE, virtual reality-based progressive resistance training; ORH, oculus rift headset; LMS, leap motion sensor; VR, virtual reality; CG, control group; LLLT, low-level laser therapy; TG, strength training associated with placebo LLLT; TLG, strength training associated with active LLLT; BS, blood sample; HGS, hand grip strength; GS, gait speed; BIA, biological impedance analysis; OA, older adult; YA, young adult; SUS, system usability scale; 6-MWT, 6-min walk test; SEMG, isokinetic protocol in isokinetic dynamometry; 1-RM, 1-repetition maximum; STS, strength training session.

Table 6.
General overview of papers focused on rehabilitation with virtual reality and laser therapy in sarcopenia.

3.1.2.2 Electrostimulation included whole-body vibration

It is well-known, from previous studies, that electrostimulation can favor the increase of muscle fibers thus improving MS, MQ, and PP and today confirmed in different works [51]. In 2016, Wittman et al. [52] and then Klemmer et al. [53–55] evaluated the parameters linked to sarcopenia and the WB-EMS effects, according to sex: the FORMOsA trial was conducted on women and the FranSO trial was conducted on men (**Table 7**).

The FORMOsA study concluded that the WB-EMS did not improve MS or PP nor decrease the fat mass, compared to the conventional physical activity [52], but it improved muscle mass. For this reason, it is advisable to use it in cases where the patient is unable to perform conventional resistance training [52, 53]. The FranSO study, on the other hand, showed that in men WB-EMS succeeded in increasing muscle mass and lowering fat mass (in sarcopenic obesity), confirming its use in the case of older people unable to move or unmotivated [54, 55].

To understand the effects of EMS intervention, Nishikawa et al. [56] made three measurements over a period of 12 weeks; then the results were compared with SEMG. Although their conclusions were closely related to a short group of individuals with the locomotive syndrome, the results suggested that EMS was able to increase MS and MQ. However, further studies would have to be performed [56] to obtain more conclusive results.

In the article by Jandova et al. [57], the EMS activity was completed in lumbar multifidus (LM) and vastus lateralis (VL). The results suggested an increase in muscle mass and mobility.

Author, year, country	Study design	Sample Mean Age ± SD	Technologies employed	Data collected/performed measurement	Session modality
Wittmann et al., 2016; Germany [52] **I** & Kemmler et al., 2016; Germany [53] **II**	RCS	75 SC-D women with MetS • WB-EMS: 77.3 ± 4.9 • WB-EMS&P: 76.4 ± 2.9 • CG: 77.4 ± 4.9	WB-EMS equipment (miha bodytec®, Gersthofen, Germany).	**I** *POP*: Change of the MetS Z-score. *SOP*: WC, MAP, TGs, FPG, HDL-C. **II** *POP*: Change in sarcopenia Z-score (EWGSOP). *SOP*: Change TBF from baseline to 26 weeks follow-up, HGS, GS, SMI.	Stratified for age, randomly assigned to: (a) n = 25 WB-EMS; (b) n = 25 WB-EMS&P and (c) n = 25 non-training CG. 6 months.
Kemmler et al., 2017; Germany [54] **I** & Kemmler et al., 2018; Germany [55] **II**	RCS	100 SC-D men with MetS: • WB-EMS: 77.1 ± 4.3 • WB-EMS&P: 78.1 ± 5.1 • CG: 76.9 ± 5.1	WB-EMS equipment (miha bodytec®, Gersthofen, Germany).	**I** *POP*: Change of the sarcopenia Z-score (FNIH criteria). *SOP*: (at baseline and after 16 weeks): TBF, SMI refers to FNIH, HGS. **II** *POP*: Changes in TBF. *SOP*: (from baseline to 16 weeks' follow-up): Changes in: TF, WC, TOT. cholesterol/HDL, cholesterol ratio, TAG.	Stratified for age, they were randomly assigned to: (a) n = 33 WB-EMS; (b) n = 33 WB-EMS&P and (c) n = 34 non-training CG. 16 weeks.
Nishikawa et al., 2019; Japan [56]	RCT	19 older women divided in: IG: n = 10; age = 75.6 ± 3.7 years; CG: n = 9; age = 77.3 ± 3.9 years.	Multi-channel SEMG (ELSCH064RS3; OT Bioelettronica, Torino, Italy); EMS.	Antropometric data and comparison with the two-step test and 25-question risk assessment between two group.	A portable EMS device to stimulate the bilateral quadriceps muscles for 8 weeks (23 minutes/5 days/week). Measurements were made at baseline, 8 weeks, and 12 weeks:
Jandova et al., 2020, Italy [57]	CSS	16 HOV of which NMES = 8, 69.3 ± 3.2 years and CG = 8, 68.0 ± 2.3 years.	NMES (Genesy 1200Pro; Globus Srl, Cologne, Italy); Muscle ultrasound.	*FT*: TUG, FTSST, VL muscle architecture, MT, PA, FL, along with VL-CSA, LM-CSA before and after by ultrasound.	3 times/week for 8 weeks.
Wu et al., 2020; China [58]	SR&M	223 participants in 7 papers: 5 with WB-VT, while 2 with L-VT.	WB-VT and L-VT	Muscle mass, muscle strength, or physical function.	8–20 minutes/12–60 Hz in L-VT; 15 minutes/300 Hz in WB-VT; 1–3 times/week for 8–12 weeks.

Author, year, country	Study design	Sample Mean Age ± SD	Technologies employed	Data collected/performed measurement	Session modality
Šarabon et al., 2020; Austria, Slovenia [59]	SR&M of RCT	2017 participants with RT, 606 with WBV, and 192 with EMS. Pooled mean age: 73.5 ± 4.8.	RT, WBV, and EMS.	(a) baseline and post-intervention mean and SD; (b) baseline demographics (c) intervention characteristics.	Typical time of intervention was 12 weeks (28) some shorter (12) and others longer (23).
Yamazaki et al., 2020; Japan [60]	CSS	64 Older adults: • NLMM (n = 51):70.6 ± 3.4 • LMM (n = 13):71.5 ± 1.9	DXA (Lunar DPX, Madison, WI, USA), SYNAPSE (Fujifilm Medical Co., Ltd, Tokyo, Japan).	Anthropometric measurements and RPW variables at 30, 60, and 240 Hz.	Measurement time was 30s, divided into two intervals of 15 s each. VS applied to the users during the last 15 s.

CSS, cross-sectional study; RCT, randomized control trials; RCS, randomized control study; MetS, metabolic syndrome; SC-D, sarcopenic community-dwelling; POP, primary outcome parameter; SOP, secondary outcome parameter; SR&M, systematic review & metanalysis; HGS, hand-grip strength; GS, gait speed; SMI, skeletal muscle mass index; EMS, electromyostimulation; DXA, dual-energy X-ray absorptiometry; WB-EMS, whole-body electromyostimulation; NMES, neuromuscular electrical stimulation; SEMG, surface electromyography; WB-EMS&P, whole-body electromyostimulation and protein supplementation; WC, waist circumference; WB-VT, whole-body vibration therapy; IG, intervention group; CG, control group; FT, functional tests; CWBV, continuous whole-body vibration; IWBV, intermittent whole-body vibration; BPP, bench press power; VJ, vertical jump (height); MAP, mean arterial pressure; TGs, triglycerides; FPG, fasting plasma glucose; HDL-C, high-density lipoprotein cholesterol; WPS, whey protein supplementation; TBF, total body fat mass; TF, trunk fat mass; TAG, triglycerides; HOV, healthy older volunteer; TUG, timed up and go test; FTSST, five times sit-to-stand test; MT, muscle thickness; PA, pennation angle; FL, fiber length; LM, lumbar multifidus; VL, vastus lateralis; VL-CSA, LM cross-sectional area; LM-CSA, LM cross-sectional area; RPW, relative proprioceptive weighting ratio VS, vibratory stimulation.

Table 7.
General overview of papers focused on electrostimulation and whole-body vibration as a sarcopenia rehabilitation tool.

On the other hand, vibration therapy (VT) was considered a close relative of EMS and showed the potential to improve MS and PP in sarcopenic older adults [58].

Initially, whole-body vibration was tested both on Asiatic and European middle-aged and older postmenopausal women [61]. Later, other studies tried to determine the optimal rate of frequency per time [62]; patients were enrolled if the diagnosis of sarcopenia was assessed by skeletal mass index. Therefore, there were some discrepancies due to the type of population and the criteria used to establish the diagnosis of sarcopenia, the point of stimulation, the type of exercises, and the measurements [58, 61]. It was compared [59] RT, WBV, and EMS and concluded that the combined use of the three techniques had the capability to improve MS and functional performance. However, more studies would be necessary to obtain more evidence that the combined use of EMS, RT, and WBV is effective in improving MS [59]. In the same year, Wu et al. [58] published a systematic review and meta-analysis showing the efficacy of WBV in improving sarcopenia and important results demonstrating an increase in MS, MQ, and PP after treatment.

Finally, Yamazaki et al. evaluated proprioception in pre-sarcopenia in a group of 64 patients [60]. However, a limitation of the study was the absence of the diagnosis of sarcopenia. Nevertheless, the results suggested that the proprioception could be linked to the decline of lower leg skeletal muscle spindles in older adults with lower muscle mass.

3.1.3 New-born technologies (not yet been tested)

Addante et al. [63] proposed new wearable devices incorporating the Arduino software to gain HGS, GS, and EMG data at the same time. Data acquisition was possible through the activation of a mobile application linked to the REST server, which was connected with the PostgreSQL database stored on a web application.

Concurrently, McGrath et al. [6] proposed a new dynamometer. It integrates the basic functionalities of any dynamometer with those of an accelerometer allowing a doubling of the features measured, obtaining a complete evaluation of the muscular capacities, integrating the parameters of MS, MQ, and PP, but only of the upper limbs.

Given the functional connection between brain activity and muscles driving the whole gait cycle, Gennaro et al. [64] proposed a mobile wireless recording device of brain activity combined with several other body behavioral variables [28, 64]. Through statistical methods based on blind source separation, they managed to segregate non-cerebral/artefactual sources from cerebral sources of activity: this system is called *"mobile brain/body imaging"* (MoBI) [64]. The obtained data were founded on coupled EEG-EMG analysis, in an interval from 0 to 1 named *"cortico-muscular coherence"* (CMC) [28, 64].

Friedrich et al. [65] introduced the MyoRobot technology (a full description is available on the biomechatronic platform [66]) designed for assessing the pathophysiologic mechanisms of muscle biomechanics. Nowadays, the technology is still being tested.

4. Discussion and conclusions

Sarcopenia is a disease that cannot be underestimated, given the impact it has on out-patient or hospitalized patients: complications, length of hospitalization, mortality, and possible problems that may occur in everyday life. In order to define target strategies or personalized therapies against sarcopenia, the diagnosis in older sarcopenic patients should be achieved through qualitative and quantitative measurements of muscle loss. Such measurements could be facilitated by the use, during hospitalization, of wearable devices capable of providing important data in a very short period of time.

In order to assess the reliability of the novel technologies proposed, a comparison on homogeneous populations should be made between the parameters obtained by using the second EWGSOP guidelines instructions and the parameters acquired through the technologies applied. Thereafter, it will be possible to define a diagnostic algorithm that would be able:

- To distinguish pre-sarcopenia from sarcopenia and severe sarcopenia, as defined by the first EWGSOP guidelines;

- On the basis of the MQ, MS, and PP parameters defined by the second EWGSOP guidelines, to build pre-sarcopenia cut-offs through the use of low-cost, safe, and useful technologies to assess pre-sarcopenia.

In conclusion, the proposed technologies are: (a) accelerometer and actigraph technology in wearable inertial sensors (**Table 1**), focused on sleep quality and loss of muscle strength, and physical activity in older adults related to PP assessment; (b) EMG for diagnostic purposes (**Table 2**); (c) JM (**Table 3**), (d) a short overview about the correlation between the PhA and muscle loss (**Table 4**); (e) a new frontier of virtual reality (**Table 6**) designed for rehabilitation programs for sarcopenic patients; (f) EMS and WBV (**Table 7**) technologies that are being studied for rehabilitation for pre-sarcopenia and sarcopenia; (g) IoT technologies, dynamometer, MoBI, and Myorobot Fiber System, which have not been yet evaluated on patients, and tools and software proposed and already tested (**Table 5**) (cfr. 3.1.3).

Devices promoting active aging could be used to design rehabilitation and prevention programs in severe sarcopenic and pre-sarcopenic patients, respectively. It would be desirable that these devices were available in hospitals, occupational medicine physicians' offices, or at general practitioner's surgeries.

Acknowledgements

I would like to thank Chiara Di Giorgio for her cooperation in the revision and the English translation of the manuscript.

Author contributions

Data acquisition: Letizia Lorusso and Luigi Esposito.
Analysis and interpretation of data: Letizia Lorusso.
The manuscript was approved and agreed on by Grazia D'Onofrio, Daniele Sancarlo, and Letizia Lorusso.

Conflict of interest

The authors have no conflicts of interest to declare.

Sarcopenia: Technological Advances in Measurement and Rehabilitation
DOI: http://dx.doi.org/10.5772/intechopen.101278

Author details

Letizia Lorusso[1], Luigi Esposito[2], Daniele Sancarlo[2] and Grazia D'Onofrio[3*]

1 Innovation and Research Unit, IRCCS - Fondazione Casa Sollievo della Sofferenza, San Giovanni Rotondo, Foggia, Italy

2 Complex Unit of Geriatrics, Department of Medical Sciences, IRCCS - Fondazione Casa Sollievo della Sofferenza, San Giovanni Rotondo, Foggia, Italy

3 Clinical Psychological Service, Health Department, IRCCS - Fondazione Casa Sollievo della Sofferenza, San Giovanni Rotondo, Foggia, Italy

*Address all correspondence to: g.donofrio@operapadrepio.it

IntechOpen

References

[1] ICD-10-CM Codes. 2021-2022 [Internet]. Available from: https://www.icd10data.com/ICD10CM/Codes/M00-M99/M60-M63/M62-/M62.84

[2] Anker SD, Morley JE, von Haehling S. Welcome to the ICD-10 code for sarcopenia. Journal of Cachexia, Sarcopenia and Muscle. 2016;7:512-514. DOI: 10.1002/jcsm.12147

[3] Vellas B, Fielding RA, Bens C, Bernabei R, Cawthon PM, Cederholm T, et al. Implications of ICD-10 for sarcopenia clinical practice and clinical trials: Report by the International Conference on Frailty and Sarcopenia Research Task Force. The Journal of Frailty & Aging. 2018;7(1):2-9. DOI: 10.14283/jfa.2017.30

[4] Cruz-Jentoft AJ, Bahat G, Bauer J, Boirie Y, Bruyère O, Cederholm T, et al. Sarcopenia: Revised European consensus on definition and diagnosis. Age and Ageing. 2019;48(1):16-31. DOI: 10.1093/ageing/afy169 [Erratum in: Age Ageing 2019;48(4):601]

[5] Cruz-Jentoft AJ, Baeyens JP, Bauer JM, Boirie Y, Cederholm T, Landi F, et al. Sarcopenia: European consensus on definition and diagnosis: Report of the European Working Group on Sarcopenia in Older People. Age and Ageing. 2010;39(4):412-423. DOI: 10.1093/ageing/afq034

[6] McGrath R, Tomkinson GR, Clark BC, Cawthon PM, Cesari M, Al Snih S, et al. Assessing additional characteristics of muscle function with digital handgrip dynamometry and accelerometry: Framework for a novel handgrip strength protocol. Journal of the American Medical Directors Association. 2021;22(11):2313-2318. DOI: 10.1016/j.jamda.2021.05.033

[7] Heymsfield SB, Gonzalez MC, Lu J, Jia G, Zheng J. Skeletal muscle mass and quality: Evolution of modern measurement concepts in the context of sarcopenia. The Proceedings of the Nutrition Society. 2015;74(4):355-366. DOI: 10.1017/S0029665115000129

[8] Fried LP, Tangen CM, Walston J, Newman AB, Hirsch C, Gottdiener J, et al. Cardiovascular Health Study Collaborative Research Group. Frailty in older adults: Evidence for a phenotype. The Journals of Gerontology. Series A, Biological Sciences and Medical Sciences. 2001;56(3):M146-M156. DOI: 10.1093/gerona/56.3.m146

[9] Institute, Ottawa, Hospital e Research, «NOSGEN.pdf». Copyright 2021 [Internet]. Available from: http://www.ohri.ca/programs/clinical_epidemiology/nosgen.pdf

[10] Foong YC, Chherawala N, Aitken D, Scott D, Winzenberg T, Jones G. Accelerometer-determined physical activity, muscle mass, and leg strength in community-dwelling older adults. Journal of Cachexia, Sarcopenia and Muscle. 2016;7(3):275-283. DOI: 10.1002/jcsm.12065

[11] Rejeski WJ, Walkup MP, Fielding RA, King AC, Manini T, Marsh AP, et al. Evaluating accelerometry thresholds for detecting changes in levels of moderate physical activity and resulting major mobility disability. The Journals of Gerontology. Series A, Biological Sciences and Medical Sciences. 2018;73(5):660-667. DOI: 10.1093/gerona/glx132

[12] Pana A, Sourtzi P, Kalokairinou A, Pastroudis A, Chatzopoulos ST, Velonaki VS. Association between muscle strength and sleep quality and duration among middle-aged and older adults: A systematic review. European Geriatric Medicine. 2021;12(1):27-44. DOI: 10.1007/s41999-020-00399-8

[13] Zytnick D, Kumar GS, Folta SC, Reid KF, Tybor D, Chomitz VR. Wearable activity monitor use is associated with the aerobic physical activity guidelines and walking among older adults. American Journal of Health Promotion. 2021;**35**(5):679-687. DOI: 10.1177/0890117120985834

[14] Kim JK, Bae MN, Lee KB, Hong SG. Identification of patients with sarcopenia using gait parameters based on inertial sensors. Sensors. 2021;**21**(5):1786. DOI: 10.3390/s21051786

[15] Dasenbrock L, Heinks A, Schwenk M, Bauer JM. Technology-based measurements for screening, monitoring and preventing frailty. Zeitschrift für Gerontologie und Geriatrie. 2016;**49**(7):581-595. DOI: 10.1007/s00391-016-1129-7

[16] Smith MT, McCrae CS, Cheung J, Martin JL, Harrod CG, Heald JL, et al. Use of actigraphy for the evaluation of sleep disorders and circadian rhythm sleep-wake disorders: An American Academy of Sleep Medicine Clinical Practice Guideline. Journal of Clinical Sleep Medicine. 2018;**14**(7):1231-1237. DOI: 10.5664/jcsm.7230

[17] Swiecicka A, Piasecki M, Stashuk DW, Ireland A, Jones DA, Rutter MK, et al. Frailty phenotype and frailty index are associated with distinct neuromuscular electrophysiological characteristics in men. Experimental Physiology. 2019;**104**(8):1154-1161. DOI: 10.1113/EP087579

[18] Bunout D, Barrera G, Hirsch S, Jimenez T, de la Maza MP. Association between activity energy expenditure and peak oxygen consumption with sarcopenia. BMC Geriatrics. 2018;**18**(1):298. DOI: 10.1186/s12877-018-0993-y

[19] CamNtech Ltd. Inc. 2020 [Internet]. Available from: https://www.camntech.com/

[20] Viecelli C, Graf D, Aguayo D, Hafen E, Füchslin RM. Using smartphone accelerometer data to obtain scientific mechanical-biological descriptors of resistance exercise training. PLoS One. 2020;**15**(7):e0235156. DOI: 10.1371/journal.pone.0235156

[21] Martineau LC, Gardiner PF. Skeletal muscle is sensitive to the tension-time integral but not to the rate of change of tension, as assessed by mechanically induced signaling. Journal of Biomechanics. 2002;**35**(5):657-663. DOI: 10.1016/s0021-9290(01)00249-4

[22] Lessard SJ, MacDonald TL, Pathak P, Han MS, Coffey VG, Edge J, et al. JNK regulates muscle remodeling via myostatin/SMAD inhibition. Nature Communications. 2018;**9**(1):3030. DOI: 10.1038/s41467-018-05439-3

[23] McPherron AC, Lawler AM, Lee SJ. Regulation of skeletal muscle mass in mice by a new TGF-beta superfamily member. Nature. 1997;**387**(6628):83-90. DOI: 10.1038/387083a0

[24] Lee SJ, McPherron AC. Regulation of myostatin activity and muscle growth. Proceedings of the National Academy of Sciences of the United States of America. 2001;**98**(16):9306-9311. DOI: 10.1073/pnas.151270098

[25] Burd NA, Andrews RJ, West DW, Little JP, Cochran AJ, Hector AJ, et al. Muscle time under tension during resistance exercise stimulates differential muscle protein sub-fractional synthetic responses in men. The Journal of Physiology. 2012;**590**(2):351-362. DOI: 10.1113/jphysiol.2011.221200

[26] Habenicht R, Ebenbichler G, Bonato P, Kollmitzer J, Ziegelbecker S, Unterlerchner L, et al. Age-specific differences in the time-frequency representation of surface electromyographic data recorded during

a submaximal cyclic back extension exercise: A promising biomarker to detect early signs of sarcopenia. Journal of Neuroengineering and Rehabilitation. 2020;**17**(1):8. DOI: 10.1186/s12984-020-0645-2

[27] Marshall RN, Morgan PT, Martinez-Valdes E, Breen L. Quadriceps muscle electromyography activity during physical activities and resistance exercise modes in younger and older adults. Experimental Gerontology. 2020;**136**:110965. DOI: 10.1016/j.exger.2020.110965

[28] Gennaro F, Maino P, Kaelin-Lang A, Bock K, Bruin ED. Corticospinal control of human locomotion as a new determinant of age-related sarcopenia: An exploratory study. Journal of Clinical Medicine. 2020;**9**(3):720. DOI: 10.3390/jcm9030720

[29] Hu CH, Yang CC, Tu SJ, Huang IJ, Ganbat D, Guo LY. Characteristics of the electrophysiological properties of neuromuscular motor units and its adaptive strategy response in lower extremity muscles for seniors with pre-sarcopenia: A preliminary study. International Journal of Environmental Research and Public Health. 2021;**18**(6):3063. DOI: 10.3390/ijerph18063063

[30] Buehring B, Krueger D, Fidler E, Gangnon R, Heiderscheit B, Binkley N. Reproducibility of jumping mechanography and traditional measures of physical and muscle function in older adults. Osteoporosis International. 2015;**26**(2):819-825. DOI: 10.1007/s00198-014-2983-z

[31] Taani MH, Kovach CR, Buehring B. Muscle mechanography: A novel method to measure muscle function in older adults. Research in Gerontological Nursing. 2017;**10**(1):17-24. DOI: 10.3928/19404921-20161209-03

[32] Dietzel R, Felsenberg D, Armbrecht G. Mechanography

performance tests and their association with sarcopenia, falls and impairment in the activities of daily living—A pilot cross-sectional study in 293 older adults. Journal of Musculoskeletal & Neuronal Interactions. 2015;**15**(3):249-256

[33] Siglinsky E, Krueger D, Ward RE, Caserotti P, Strotmeyer ES, Harris TB, et al. Effect of age and sex on jumping mechanography and other measures of muscle mass and function. Journal of Musculoskeletal & Neuronal Interactions. 2015;**15**(4):301-308

[34] Hannam K, Hartley A, Clark EM, Aihie Sayer A, Tobias JH, Gregson CL. Feasibility and acceptability of using jumping mechanography to detect early components of sarcopenia in community-dwelling older women. Journal of Musculoskeletal & Neuronal Interactions. 2017;**17**(3):246-257

[35] Minett MM, Binkley TL, Holm RP, Runge M, Specker BL. Feasibility and effects on muscle function of an exercise program for older adults. Medicine and Science in Sports and Exercise. 2020;**52**(2):441-448. DOI: 10.1249/MSS.0000000000002152

[36] Alvero-Cruz JR, Brikis M, Chilibeck P, Frings-Meuthen P, Vico Guzmán JF, Mittag U, et al. Age-related decline in vertical jumping performance in masters track and field athletes: Concomitant influence of body composition. Frontiers in Physiology. 2021;**12**:643649. DOI: 10.3389/fphys.2021.643649

[37] Wiegmann S, Felsenberg D, Armbrecht G, Dietzel R. Longitudinal changes in muscle power compared to muscle strength and mass. Journal of Musculoskeletal & Neuronal Interactions. 2021;**21**(1):13-25

[38] Kilic MK, Kizilarslanoglu MC, Arik G, Bolayir B, Kara O, Dogan Varan H, et al. Association of bioelectrical impedance

analysis-derived phase angle and sarcopenia in older adults. Nutrition in Clinical Practice. 2017;**32**(1):103-109. DOI: 10.1177/0884533616664503

[39] Ceniccola GD, Castro MG, Piovacari SMF, Horie LM, Corrêa FG, Barrere APN, et al. Current technologies in body composition assessment: Advantages and disadvantages. Nutrition. 2019;**62**:25-31. DOI: 10.1016/j.nut.2018.11.028

[40] Pessoa DF, de Branco FMS, Dos Reis AS, Limirio LS, Borges LP, Barbosa CD, et al. Association of phase angle with sarcopenia and its components in physically active older women. Aging Clinical and Experimental Research. 2020;**32**(8):1469-1475. DOI: 10.1007/s40520-019-01325-0

[41] Rosas-Carrasco O, Ruiz-Valenzuela RE, López-Teros MT. Phase angle cut-off points and their association with sarcopenia and frailty in adults of 50-64 years old and older adults in Mexico City. Frontiers in Medicine. 2021;**8**:617126. DOI: 10.3389/fmed.2021.617126

[42] Beveridge LA, Price RJG, Burton LA, Witham MD, Struthers AD, Sumukadas D. Acceptability and feasibility of magnetic femoral nerve stimulation in older, functionally impaired patients. BMC Research Notes. 2018;**11**(1):394. DOI: 10.1186/s13104-018-3493-4

[43] Lera L, Angel B, Márquez C, Saguez R, Albala C. Software for the diagnosis of sarcopenia in community-dwelling older adults: Design and validation study. JMIR Medical Informatics. 2020;**8**(4):e13657. DOI: 10.2196/13657

[44] Bachasson D, Ayaz AC, Mosso J, Canal A, Boisserie JM, Araujo ECA, et al. Lean regional muscle volume estimates using explanatory bioelectrical models in healthy subjects and patients with muscle wasting. Journal of Cachexia, Sarcopenia and Muscle. 2021;**12**(1):39-51. DOI: 10.1002/jcsm.12656

[45] Coelho-Junior HJ, Marzetti E, Picca A, Cesari M, Uchida MC, Calvani R. Protein intake and frailty: A matter of quantity, quality, and timing. Nutrients. 2020;**12**(10):2915. DOI: 10.3390/nu12102915

[46] Agostini F, Bernetti A, Di Giacomo G, Viva MG, Paoloni M, Mangone M, et al. Rehabilitative good practices in the treatment of sarcopenia: A narrative review. American Journal of Physical Medicine & Rehabilitation. 2021;**100**(3):280-287. DOI: 10.1097/PHM.0000000000001572

[47] Tuena C, Pedroli E, Trimarchi PD, Gallucci A, Chiappini M, Goulene K, et al. Usability issues of clinical and research applications of virtual reality in older people: A systematic review. Frontiers in Human Neuroscience. 2020;**14**:93. DOI: 10.3389/fnhum.2020.00093

[48] Scott RA, Callisaya ML, Duque G, Ebeling PR, Scott D. Assistive technologies to overcome sarcopenia in ageing. Maturitas. 2018;**112**:78-84. DOI: 10.1016/j.maturitas.2018.04.003

[49] Toma RL, Vassão PG, Assis L, Antunes HK, Renno AC. Low level laser therapy associated with a strength training program on muscle performance in elderly women: A randomized double blind control study. Lasers in Medical Science. 2016;**31**(6):1219-1229. DOI: 10.1007/s10103-016-1967-y

[50] Chen GB, Lin CW, Huang HY, Wu YJ, Su HT, Sun SF, et al. Using virtual reality-based rehabilitation in sarcopenic older adults in rural health care facilities—A quasi-experimental study. Journal of Aging and Physical

Activity. 2021;**29**(5):866-877. DOI: 10.1123/japa.2020-0222

[51] Evangelista AL, Alonso AC, Ritti-Dias RM, Barros BM, de Souza CR, Braz TV, et al. Effects of whole body electrostimulation associated with body weight training on functional capacity and body composition in inactive older people. Frontiers in Physiology. 2021;**12**:638936. DOI: 10.3389/fphys.2021.638936 [Erratum in: Front Physiol 2021;12:694855; Front Physiol 2021;12:714782]

[52] Wittmann K, Sieber C, von Stengel S, Kohl M, Freiberger E, Jakob F, et al. Impact of whole body electromyostimulation on cardiometabolic risk factors in older women with sarcopenic obesity: The randomized controlled FORMOsA-sarcopenic obesity study. Clinical Interventions in Aging. 2016;**11**:1697-1706. DOI: 10.2147/CIA.S116430

[53] Kemmler W, Teschler M, Weissenfels A, Bebenek M, von Stengel S, Kohl M, et al. Whole-body electromyostimulation to fight sarcopenic obesity in community-dwelling older women at risk. Results of the randomized controlled FORMOsA-sarcopenic obesity study. Osteoporosis International. 2016;**27**(11):3261-3270. DOI: 10.1007/s00198-016-3662-z

[54] Kemmler W, Weissenfels A, Teschler M, Willert S, Bebenek M, Shojaa M, et al. Whole-body electromyostimulation and protein supplementation favorably affect sarcopenic obesity in community-dwelling older men at risk: The randomized controlled FranSO study. Clinical Interventions in Aging. 2017;**12**:1503-1513. DOI: 10.2147/CIA.S137987

[55] Kemmler W, Kohl M, Freiberger E, Sieber C, von Stengel S. Effect of whole-body electromyostimulation and/or protein supplementation on obesity and cardiometabolic risk in older men with sarcopenic obesity: The randomized controlled FranSO trial. BMC Geriatrics. 2018;**18**(1):70. DOI: 10.1186/s12877-018-0759-6

[56] Nishikawa Y, Watanabe K, Kawade S, Takahashi T, Kimura H, Maruyama H, et al. The effect of a portable electrical muscle stimulation device at home on muscle strength and activation patterns in locomotive syndrome patients: A randomized control trial. Journal of Electromyography and Kinesiology. 2019;**45**:46-52. DOI: 10.1016/j.jelekin.2019.02.007

[57] Jandova T, Narici MV, Steffl M, Bondi D, D'Amico M, Pavlu D, et al. Muscle hypertrophy and architectural changes in response to eight-week neuromuscular electrical stimulation training in healthy older people. Life (Basel). 2020;**10**(9):184. DOI: 10.3390/life10090184

[58] Wu S, Ning HT, Xiao SM, Hu MY, Wu XY, Deng HW, et al. Effects of vibration therapy on muscle mass, muscle strength and physical function in older adults with sarcopenia: A systematic review and meta-analysis. European Review of Aging and Physical Activity. 2020;**17**:14. DOI: 10.1186/s11556-020-00247-5

[59] Šarabon N, Kozinc Ž, Löfler S, Hofer C. Resistance exercise, electrical muscle stimulation, and whole-body vibration in older adults: Systematic review and meta-analysis of randomized controlled trials. Journal of Clinical Medicine. 2020;**9**(9):2902. DOI: 10.3390/jcm9092902

[60] Yamazaki K, Ito T, Sakai Y, Nishio R, Ito Y, Morita Y. Postural sway during local vibratory stimulation for proprioception in elderly individuals with pre-sarcopenia. Physical Therapy Research. 2020;**23**(2):149-152. DOI: 10.1298/ptr.E10001

[61] Boggild MK, Tomlinson G, Erlandson MC, Szabo E, Giangregorio LM, Craven BC, et al. Effects of whole-body vibration therapy on distal tibial myotendinous density and volume: A randomized controlled trial in postmenopausal women. JBMR Plus. 2018;**3**(5):e10120. DOI: 10.1002/jbm4.10120

[62] Wei N, Pang MY, Ng SS, Ng GY. Optimal frequency/time combination of whole-body vibration training for improving muscle size and strength of people with age-related muscle loss (sarcopenia): A randomized controlled trial. Geriatrics & Gerontology International. 2017;**17**(10):1412-1420. DOI: 10.1111/ggi.12878

[63] Addante F, Gaetani F, Patrono L, Sancarlo D, Sergi I, Vergari G. An innovative AAL system based on IoT technologies for patients with sarcopenia. Sensors. 2019;**19**(22):4951. DOI: 10.3390/s19224951

[64] Gennaro F, de Bruin ED. Assessing brain-muscle connectivity in human locomotion through mobile brain/body imaging: Opportunities, pitfalls, and future directions. Frontiers in Public Health. 2018;**6**:39. DOI: 10.3389/fpubh.2018.00039

[65] Friedrich O, Haug M, Reischl B, Prölß G, Kiriaev L, Head SI, et al. Single muscle fibre biomechanics and biomechatronics—The challenges, the pitfalls and the future. The International Journal of Biochemistry & Cell Biology. 2019;**114**:105563. DOI: 10.1016/j.biocel.2019.105563

[66] FAU-Friedrich-Alexander-Universitat Erlangen Nurnberg. Medical Bio-Technology. 2021 [Internet]. Available from: https://www.mbt.tf.fau.de/research/research-groups/opto-biomechatronics/the-myorobot-prototype/

Chapter 5

Attenuating Cancer Cachexia-Prolonging Life

Charles Lambert

Abstract

Death by cancer cachexia is dependent on the time allotted to cancer to cause muscle and fat wasting. If clinicians, nurses, researchers can prolong the life of a cancer patient other therapeutic interventions such as radiation and chemotherapy may be given the time to work and rid the cancer patient of tumors and save lives. Three areas by which cancer induces cachexia is through impaired insulin-like growth factor signaling, elevations in the proinflammatory cytokines TNF-α and IL-6 and subsequent reductions in muscle protein synthesis and increases in muscle protein degradation. Therefore, it is important to augment the IGF-1 signaling, block TNF-α and IL-6 in cancer cachexia and in other ways augment muscle protein synthesis or decrease muscle protein degradation. Ghrelin like growth hormone secretagogues, monoclonal antibodies to TNF-α and IL-6, testosterone, and anabolic steroids, the beta 2 agonist albuterol, resistance exercise, and creatine monohydrate (with resistance exercise) are beneficial in increasing muscle protein synthesis and/or reducing muscle protein breakdown. With these muscle augmenting agents/interventions, the duration that a cancer patient lives is prolonged so that radiation and chemotherapy as well as emerging technologies can rid the cancer patient of cancer and save lives.

Keywords: muscle wasting, anabolism, oncology, nutrition, exercise, pharmacotherapy

1. Introduction

There are no drugs approved to treat cancer cachexia in the US. This is unfortunate and a flaw, I believe, in the FDAs criteria for cancer cachexia drug approval in the United States [1]. Their criterion measure has been an improvement in function. This variable depends on the nervous system in addition to skeletal muscle because they are functional in nature. Cachexia, by definition is the loss of skeletal muscle and adipose tissue. Drugs designed to affect skeletal muscle have little and probably no effect on the nervous system. As such, the FDA should remove the functional requirement or make functional training along with drug administration a requirement in phase I, II and III studies. As it is, all drugs anabolic to skeletal muscle will likely fail a functional test since they have no effect, without functional exercise, on the nervous system.

With this short coming of the approval process in mind, other measures must be taken to attenuate cachexia with the intent of allowing more time for chemotherapeutic agents and radiation therapy to exert their tumor killing activity. It is indeed a matter of time for cachectic cancer patients; the more time they have, the better the outcome with the goal to be to cure cancer for those individuals suffering from cancer cachexia and save lives. Off-label use of drugs that are approved for other conditions would appear to be a very important action to take for clinicians to this end. For example, the use of monoclonal antibodies for IL-6 and TNF-α which are approved for other indications would appear beneficial in treating many cancers as these proinflammatory cytokines are secreted during cancer-inflammation mediated by these cytokines wreaks havoc on the patient. In addition, IL-6 and TNF-α are directly related to muscle catabolism in models of cancer cachexia [2, 3]. Hypermetabolism is another manifestation of cancer cachexia [4]. Drugs that block the action of epinephrine (a catecholamine) would act to reduce metabolic rate and slow the rate of muscle wasting [5]. The drug propranolol blocks both beta 1 and beta 2 receptors metabolic rate. This is just one example of a drug that could reduce hypermetabolism of cachexia. A third factor, although taboo especially in the sporting world, is the use of anabolic agents to stimulate muscle protein synthesis [6–8] in the face of reduced muscle protein synthesis, and elevated muscle protein breakdown. Thus, the off-label use of anabolic steroids, testosterone, and growth hormone secretagogues should be explored although some these agents are not FDA approved. For example, anamorelin was found to be safe and effective in increasing lean body mass through phase III trials but did not increase grip strength [9].

2. Mechanisms of IL-6 induced muscle catabolism

In one study, to date, IL-6 has been shown to reduce basal and eccentric exercise induced protein synthesis by generally well accepted mechanisms [10].

One mechanism by which IL-6 decreases muscle mass is by activating the STAT 3 pathway which causes muscle protein breakdown to acute phase proteins. An acute phase protein derived from skeletal muscle that is synthesized upon IL-6 binding in skeletal muscle and activation of the STAT 3 pathway is fibrinogen. This was reported in an experimental animal model of cancer cachexia [2]. In a subsequent study this group also reported that blocking the JAK/STAT 3 pathway inhibited skeletal muscle wasting [3]. Therefore, this is a way that IL-6 induces muscle protein breakdown also known as proteolysis.

Another mechanism described in the literature [11] is autophagy where the cells in essence eat themselves. This would be considered a second mechanism by which proteolysis is induced by IL-6.

A third mechanism by which IL-6 can induce protein breakdown is by activation of atrogin 1 (MAFBX) [12].

3. Mechanisms of TNF-α induced muscle catabolism

In a pre-clinical proof of concept study Lang et al. [13] reported that a TNF-α infusion to rats reduced the muscle protein synthesis rate (decreased by 39%) by way of reducing the mRNA to protein conversion (decreased by 39%) of both myofibrillar and sarcoplasmic proteins in the gastrocnemius muscle. The plasma TNF-α concentration was raised to 500 pg/ml in this study.

A question that remains is: is it the plasma concentration of the TNF-α that is important and/or the muscle derived TNF-α [14] that is important in the regulation of muscle protein synthesis. A similar example in skeletal muscle are the acute phase proteins which are derived from muscle such as fibrinogen.

On the muscle protein breakdown side of the muscle mass equation, Li et al. [15] reported that TNF-α utilizes the p38 MAPK pathway to cause expression of atrogin-1/MAFBX in skeletal muscle. This activation of atrogin-1/MAFBX activates the ubiquitin-proteasome pathway for muscle protein degradation. This was confirmed when inhibitors of p38 inhibited ubiquitin conjugation activity.

4. Impairment of the IGF-1 pathway in muscle catabolism

Endogenous insulin-like growth factor-1 (IGF-1) is a very potent anabolic agent in the human body. IGF-1 is released from the liver after growth hormone (GH) stimulation of liver cells. Another form of IGF-1 (a splice variant) mechano-growth factor (MGF) is produced by the mechanical loading of skeletal muscle [16] and is released in a paracrine/autocrine fashion and is also a potent anabolic agent. Lambert et al. [14] reported that the combination of chronic aerobic and resistance exercise training in humans, resulted in an upregulation in MGF mRNA in skeletal muscle.

The mechanism of action of IGF-1 in causing muscle protein synthesis is through PI3K/AKT/mTOR signaling [17]. This would also be the pathway via a common receptor by which insulin stimulates muscle protein synthesis. Interestingly, lack of basal IGF-1 signaling resulted in activation of atrogin-1 and Murf-1, two factors that induce muscle protein breakdown through the ubiquitin-proteasome pathway [17, 18]. Additionally, these authors [18] reported when basal IGF-1 levels were absent there was an activation of GSK-3B which phosphorylates and inactivates 4EBP1-a translation (protein synthesis) initiation factor. This activation of muscle protein breakdown through these two mediators resulted in myosin heavy chain 1 and 3 degradation in an animal model. In addition to causing muscle protein synthesis, IGF-1 acts to reduce muscle protein breakdown through reducing atrogin-1 and Murf-1.

In a thorough study on the effects of cancer cachexia on the IGF-1 system in skeletal muscle and plasma, Costelli et al. [19] reported that there was about a 50% reduction in muscle IGF-1 and plasma levels were also reduced. The model they used for cancer cachexia was the Yoshida AH-130 hepatoma model [19].

To summarize, IGF-1 is a potent stimulator of anabolism or muscle growth and impairing the signaling of IGF-1 results in reduced muscle protein synthesis through the PI3K/AKT/mTOR pathway as well as increased muscle protein degradation through an increase in atrogin-1 and Murf-1. Additionally, GSK-3B is activated which inhibits translation initiation by phosphorylating 4EBP-1 when IGF-1 signaling is impaired.

5. Treatment of cachexia

5.1 Resistance exercise training

Weight training or more commonly known as resistance exercise training in which an individual contracts his muscles against the force of a weight stack, free weights, or sometimes resistance bands is a way in which to increase muscle protein synthesis [20]. This bodes well for the cancer patient if they have the functional ability to undergo these types of workouts. It is well known that this increase in protein synthesis chronically will result in an increase in muscle mass. An additional benefit of exercise and likely a precursor to muscle growth is a decrease in intramuscular proinflammatory cytokine mRNAs and an increase in mechano-growth factor mRNA which is a slice variant of IGF-1.

5.2 Creatine monohydrate

An adjunct nutritional supplement to resistance training is creatine (monohydrate). Creatine when ingested in sufficient quantities, for example, 20 g/day for 5 days will elevate the intramuscular stores of creatine. This elevation of intramuscular creatine can increase the rate of phosphocreatine resynthesis in man [21]. This is by way of the reaction ATP + creatine yields PCr + ADP. Where ATP is adenosine triphosphate, PCr is phosphocreatine, and ADP is adenosine triphosphate. Creatine ingestion in the manner described above improves not only PCr resynthesis but also exercise capacity [22].

5.3 Ibuprofen and acetaminophen

It is well known that a bout of resistance training will increase muscle protein synthesis in the hours after exercise [20]. Resistance exercise also increases the muscle protein degradative cytokines IL-6 and murf-1 mRNA [23]. Resistance exercise with ibuprofen or acetaminophen ingestion blunts the IL-6 and murf-1 response to resistance exercise [23]. Cancer cachexia increases IL-6 and murf-1 leading to more protein degradation [10]. Therefore resistance exercise with acetaminophen or ibuprofen is beneficial for increasing muscle protein synthesis and decreasing muscle protein breakdown to achieve a more favorable response (increasing synthesis and decreasing breakdown = more + net protein balance; Trappe et al. [23]). This would improve the ability to accrete more muscle mass in the face of cancer cachexia. It is suggested that future clinical trials combine resistance training with acetaminophen or ibuprofen at the maximal daily dosage in cachectic cancer patients. For detailed schematic on how these analgesic agents affect protein metabolism see Trappe et al. [23].

5.4 Albuterol

In humans, Uc et al. [24] found that administration of the beta-2 agonist albuterol increased thigh cross-sectional area by 5.3% and whole-body fat free mass by 9.5% in Parkinson's patients over 14 weeks (16 mg/day). Unpublished data suggests that muscle protein synthesis is elevated by ~90% in elderly individuals with 16 mg/day over 10 days of albuterol administration (Lambert et al. unpublished observations). Albuterol would appear to be an anabolic agent that should be administered off label in cancer cachexia in clinical trials.

5.5 Anamorelin and ibutamorelin

Anamorelin is active orally, centrally penetrant, and selective agonist of the ghrelin/growth hormone secretagogue receptor-1a and was under development for the treatment of cancer cachexia and anorexia [25] (Drug Bank). It increases growth hormone (GH), insulin-like growth factor-1 (IGF-1) and insulin-like growth factor binding protein (IGFBP-3) and apparently has no side effects as testosterone administration does. It also stimulates appetite [9]. It has been shown in Phase III Clinical Trials to increase appetite, body weight, lean body mass, but not muscle strength as measured by hand grip strength [9]. The natural agonist for ghrelin/growth hormone secretagogue receptor-1a, ghrelin has a short half-life, however; anamorelin has better pharmacokinetic properties as evidenced by a more sustained delivery [26]. It is a dipepetide of molecular weight 546.716 (Drug Bank). Apparently, this drug failed in Phase III Clinical Trials due to lack of an effect on grip strength although it increased lean body mass [9]. The only side effect noted with anamorelin was a small risk of headache [26]. Anamorelin is approved for clinical use in Japan but not the US or Europe.

Ibutamorelin, like anamorelin, is another ghrelin analogue that stimulates growth hormone secretion from the pituitary and IGF-1 secretion from the liver. Svenson et al. reported that 2 months of treatment of individuals 18–50 years old with 25 mg of ibutamorelin resulted in and increase in growth hormone and IGF-1 and a significant increase in fat free mass when measured by DEXA or by a four compartment model. Basal metabolic rate was elevated at 2 weeks but not at 8 weeks. Nass et al. [27] reported that in individuals 60–81 years of age, 25 mg of ibutamorelin administered over 2 years resulted in a loss of 0.5 kg of fat free mass in placebo group but a gain of 1.1 kg in the ibutamorelin group. This was accompanied by an increase in growth hormone and IGF-1 and a reduction in LDL cholesterol of 0.14 mmol/L. Murphy et al. (1998) reported that in individuals 24–39 years of age, ibutamorelin (25 mg/day) accompanied by a 18 kcal/kg/day energy intake for 2, 14 day periods resulted in a + 2.69 nitrogen balance for the ibutamorelin group but a −8.97 for the placebo group during the last 7 days of the second 14 days, which suggests that this anabolic agent would be preventative of muscle loss with a very low energy intake. Unfortunately, ibutamorelin did not show efficacy in functional tests which are the criteria the FDA uses for cancer cachexia drugs [1] and in other conditions which induce muscle loss such as hip fracture [28]. Both anamorelin and ibutamorelin did not show functional efficacy in clinical trials. Why functional capacity improvement would be the ultimate criteria for cancer cachexia would be beyond me. Since the problem in cancer cachexia would be considered muscle wasting and not a functional problem [1]. Maybe it is time for the FDA to change their criteria for approval of safe and effective drugs which cause anabolism and prevent catabolism during cancer cachexia. Because of the FDAs short sightedness, both of these drugs (anamorelin and ibutamorelin) have been rendered the status of nutritional supplements.

5.6 Megace

Megestrol acetate (Megace) stimulates appetite, increases feeding behavior, alone-reduces lean body mass-but in combination with testosterone therapy and resistance exercise training, increases lean body mass in underweight elderly men [29]. This combination of Megace, testosterone, and resistance training may be beneficial in cancer patients. Megace alone decreased muscle mass but when combined with testosterone AND exercise resulted in a substantial increase in muscle mass in 12 weeks of training and administration [29]. It was hypothesized by the authors that Megace binds to the androgen receptor and blocks the action of testosterone. However, when combined with resistance exercise and testosterone replacement (100 mg/week) resulted in substantial muscle growth (hypertrophy). Therefore, resistance exercise, in some way acts, permissively to allows underweight elderly men to maintain muscle mass when testosterone is low and in the face of testosterone replacement to increase muscle mass. Likely, this is through the androgen receptor.

5.7 Testosterone and anabolic steroids

Testosterone and anabolic steroids are anabolic to skeletal muscle [30]. Bhasin et al. [30] illustrated the fact that testosterone is anabolic to skeletal muscle in stepwise fashion with increasing dosage. The correlation between log testosterone and lean body mass (a surrogate for muscle mass) was 0.73, a very strong correlation. Urban et al. [6] reported that the mechanism of action of testosterone, with regard to, skeletal muscle anabolism in elderly individuals with low testosterone (testosterone < 480 ng/dL), was an increase in muscle protein synthesis which appear by elevated muscle IGF-1 concentrations and to be mediated by an elevation of IGF-1 in skeletal muscle. Cancer patients in general are hypogonadal (testosterone concentrations less than 300 ng/dL; Burney et al. [31]). Therefore, the administration of testosterone or its much less androgenic (secondary side effects) analogue anabolic steroids would appear to be a logical step in the treatment of cancer cachexia which may at least partly be due to low testosterone concentrations. The only caveat is that cancers that are hormone sensitive may not be a good candidate for testosterone or anabolic steroid therapy due to possible proliferation of the tumor. Nandrolone decanoate, an intramuscular injectable anabolic steroid and oxandrolone, an oral anabolic steroid are very low in secondary side effects because of their low androgenic to anabolic ratio. They have been used in other disease populations such as HIV [7] for oxandrolone and nandrolone decanoate [8]. Thus, the utility of these drugs along with testosterone in cancer would appear unquestionable. Clinical trials using these anabolic agents in an off label fashion in multiple types of cancer is warranted.

5.8 Monoclonal antibodies

A logical step in decreasing the cachexia associated with cancer would be neutralizing circulating IL-6 and TNF-α with monoclonal antibodies.

There are many monoclonal antibodies to TNF-α FDA approved for other uses. To the best of my knowledge, there are one or a few monoclonal antibodies to IL-6 for different indications than cancer. Clearly, as discussed in a recent letter to the editor [5], this would be a very important application of monoclonal antibody technology.

6. Conclusion

Inflammation through IL-6 and TNF-α is an important mechanism by which cancer causes muscle catabolism. Reducing inflammation by exercise, non-steroidal anti-inflammatory drugs, and monoclonal antibodies would appear to be a potential strategy to curtail cancer cachexia. Also, augmenting protein synthesis by utilizing exercise, creatine monohydrate, albuterol, testosterone, and anabolic steroids would also appear to be a potential strategy to curtail cancer cachexia. Utilizing megestrol acetate would be indicated for cancer cachexia only if accompanied by testosterone replacement and exercise. The off-label oral use of albuterol is anabolic to skeletal muscle in healthy elderly individuals and future clinical trials could evaluate its utility in cancer cachexia. Ghrelin analogues, that is, growth hormone secretagogues, although not FDA approved, elevate, in pulsatile manner, growth hormone and IGF-1 concentrations and increase significantly lean body mass accrual (some studies in cancer) with few if any side effects. Therefore, these nutritional supplements are indicated for the treatment of cancer cachexia. For a depiction of Ligand-Receptor interactions discussed in this Chapter please see (**Figure 1**).

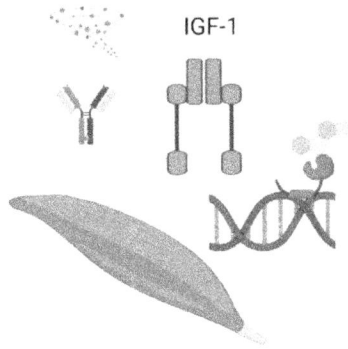

Figure 1.
A schematic representation of monoclonal antibodies and cytokines, mechanism of action of growth hormone and putative mechanism of beta-2 agonists in animals, and of testosterone and anabolic steroids on skeletal muscle.

Author details

Charles Lambert
University of California, San Diego, USA

†Address all correspondence to: clcpl368@gmail.com

IntechOpen

References

[1] Lambert CP. Should the FDA's criteria for the clinical efficacy of cachexia drugs be changed? Is ostarine safe and effective? Journal of Cachexia, Sarcopenia and Muscle. 2021;**12**(3):531-532

[2] Bonetto A, Aydogdu T, Kunzevitzky N, Guttridge DC, Khuri S, Koniaris LG, et al. STAT3 activation in skeletal muscle links muscle wasting and the acute phase response in cancer cachexia. PLoS One. 2011;**6**(7):e22538

[3] Bonetto A, Aydogdu T, Jin X, Zhang Z, Zhan R, Puzis L, et al. JAK/STAT3 pathway inhibition blocks skeletal muscle wasting downstream of IL-6 and in experimental cancer cachexia. American Journal of Physiology. Endocrinology and Metabolism. 2012;**303**(3):E410-E421

[4] Grip J, Jakobsson T, Hebert C, Klaude M, Sandstrom G, Wernerman J, et al. Lactate kinetics and mitochondrial respiration in skeletal muscle of healthy humans under influence of adrenaline. Clinical Science. 2015;**129**(4):375-384

[5] Lambert CP. Anti-cachexia therapy should target metabolism, inflammatory cytokines, and androgens in hormone-independent cancers. Journal of Cachexia, Sarcopenia and Muscle. 2021;**12**(5):1352-1353

[6] Urban RJ, Bodenburg YH, Gilkison C, Foxworth J, Coggan AR, Wolfe RR, et al. Testosterone administration to elderly men increases skeletal muscle strength and protein synthesis. The American Journal of Physiology. 1995;**269**(5 Pt 1):E820-E826

[7] Grunfeld C, Kotler DP, Dobs A, Glesby M, Bhasin S. Oxandrolone in the treatment of HIV-associated weight loss in men: A randomized, double-blind, placebo-controlled study. Journal of Acquired Immune Deficiency Syndromes. 2006;**41**(3):304-314

[8] Batterham MJ, Garsia R. A comparison of megestrol acetate, nandrolone decanoate and dietary counselling for HIV associated weight loss. International Journal of Andrology. 2001;**24**(4):232-240

[9] Temel JS, Abernethy AP, Currow DC, Friend J, Duus EM, Yan Y, et al. Anamorelin in patients with non-small-cell lung cancer and cachexia (ROMANA 1 and ROMANA 2): Results from two randomised, double-blind, phase 3 trials. The Lancet Oncology. 2016;**17**(4):519-531

[10] Hardee JP, Fix DK, Wang X, Goldsmith EC, Koh HJ, Carson JA. Systemic IL-6 regulation of eccentric contraction-induced muscle protein synthesis. American Journal of Physiology. Cell Physiology. 2018; **315**(1):C91-C103

[11] Pettersen K, Andersen S, Degen S, Tadini V, Grosjean J, Hatakeyama S, et al. Cancer cachexia associates with a systemic autophagy-inducing activity mimicked by cancer cell-derived IL-6 trans-signaling. Scientific Reports. 2017;**7**(1):2046

[12] Bonetto A, Rupert JE, Barreto R, Zimmers TA. The colon-26 carcinoma tumor-bearing mouse as a model for the study of cancer cachexia. Journal of Visualized Experiments. 2016;(117):54893. DOI: 10.3791/54893

[13] Lang CH, Frost RA, Nairn AC, MacLean DA, Vary TC. TNF-alpha impairs heart and skeletal muscle protein synthesis by altering translation initiation. American Journal of Physiology. Endocrinology and Metabolism. 2002;**282**(2):E336-E347

[14] Lambert CP, Wright NR, Finck BN, Villareal DT. Exercise but not diet-induced weight loss decreases skeletal muscle inflammatory gene expression in

frail obese elderly persons. Journal of Applied Physiology. 2008;**105**(2): 473-478

[15] Li YP, Chen Y, John J, Moylan J, Jin B, Mann DL, et al. TNF-alpha acts via p38 MAPK to stimulate expression of the ubiquitin ligase atrogin1/MAFbx in skeletal muscle. The FASEB Journal. 2005;**19**(3):362-370

[16] Hameed M, Orrell RW, Cobbold M, Goldspink G, Harridge SD. Expression of IGF-I splice variants in young and old human skeletal muscle after high resistance exercise. The Journal of Physiology. 2003;**547**(Pt 1):247-254

[17] Stitt TN, Drujan D, Clarke BA, Panaro F, Timofeyva Y, Kline WO, et al. The IGF-1/PI3K/Akt pathway prevents expression of muscle atrophy-induced ubiquitin ligases by inhibiting FOXO transcription factors. Molecular Cell. 2004;**14**(3):395-403

[18] Verhees KJ, Schols AM, Kelders MC, Op den Kamp CM, van der Velden JL, Langen RC. Glycogen synthase kinase-3beta is required for the induction of skeletal muscle atrophy. American Journal of Physiology. Cell Physiology. 2011;**301**(5):C995-C1007

[19] Costelli P, Muscaritoli M, Bossola M, Penna F, Reffo P, Bonetto A, et al. IGF-1 is downregulated in experimental cancer cachexia. American Journal of Physiology. Regulatory, Integrative and Comparative Physiology. 2006;**291**(3): R674-R683

[20] Phillips SM, Parise G, Roy BD, Tipton KD, Wolfe RR, Tamopolsky MA. Resistance-training-induced adaptations in skeletal muscle protein turnover in the fed state. Canadian Journal of Physiology and Pharmacology. 2002; **80**(11):1045-1053

[21] Greenhaff PL, Bodin K, Soderlund K, Hultman E. Effect of oral creatine supplementation on skeletal muscle phosphocreatine resynthesis. The American Journal of Physiology. 1994;**266**(5 Pt 1):E725-E730

[22] Casey A, Constantin-Teodosiu D, Howell S, Hultman E, Greenhaff PL. Creatine ingestion favorably affects performance and muscle metabolism during maximal exercise in humans. The American Journal of Physiology. 1996;**271**(1 Pt 1):E31-E37

[23] Trappe TA, Standley RA, Jemiolo B, Carroll CC, Trappe SW. Prostaglandin and myokine involvement in the cyclooxygenase-inhibiting drug enhancement of skeletal muscle adaptations to resistance exercise in older adults. American Journal of Physiology. Regulatory, Integrative and Comparative Physiology. 2013;**304**(3): R198-R205

[24] Uc EY, Lambert CP, Harik SI, Rodnitzky RL, Evans WJ. Albuterol improves response to levodopa and increases skeletal muscle mass in patients with fluctuating Parkinson disease. Clinical Neuropharmacology. 2003;**26**(4):207-212

[25] Pietra C, Takeda Y, Tazawa-Ogata N, Minami M, Yuanfeng X, Duus EM, et al. Anamorelin HCl (ONO-7643), a novel ghrelin receptor agonist, for the treatment of cancer anorexia-cachexia syndrome: Preclinical profile. Journal of Cachexia, Sarcopenia and Muscle. 2014;**5**(4):329-337

[26] Leese PT, Trang JM, Blum RA, de Groot E. An open-label clinical trial of the effects of age and gender on the pharmacodynamics, pharmacokinetics and safety of the ghrelin receptor agonist anamorelin. Clinical Pharmacology in Drug Development. 2015;**4**(2):112-120

[27] Nass R, Pezzoli SS, Oliveri MC, Patrie JT, Harrell FE Jr, Clasey JL, et al. Effects of an oral ghrelin mimetic on body composition and clinical outcomes

in healthy older adults: A randomized trial. Annals of Internal Medicine. 2008; **149**(9):601-611

[28] Bach MA, Rockwood K, Zetterberg C, Thamsborg G, Hebert R, Devogelaer JP, et al. The effects of MK-0677, an oral growth hormone secretagogue, in patients with hip fracture. Journal of the American Geriatrics Society. 2004;**52**(4):516-523

[29] Lambert CP, Sullivan DH, Freeling SA, Lindquist DM, Evans WJ. Effects of testosterone replacement and/ or resistance exercise on the composition of megestrol acetate stimulated weight gain in elderly men: A randomized controlled trial. The Journal of Clinical Endocrinology and Metabolism. 2002;**87**(5):2100-2106

[30] Bhasin S, Storer TW, Berman N, Callegari C, Clevenger B, Phillips J, et al. The effects of supraphysiologic doses of testosterone on muscle size and strength in normal men. The New England Journal of Medicine. 1996;**335**(1):1-7

[31] Burney BO, Hayes TG, Smiechowska J, Cardwell G, Papusha V, Bhargava P, et al. Low testosterone levels and increased inflammatory markers in patients with cancer and relationship with cachexia. The Journal of Clinical Endocrinology and Metabolism. 2012; **97**(5):E700-E709

Cardiac and Cancer-Associated Cachexia: Role of Exercise Training, Non-coding RNAs, and Future Perspectives

Bruno Rocha de Avila Pelozin, Luis Felipe Rodrigues, Edilamar Menezes De Oliveira and Tiago Fernandes

Abstract

Sarcopenia has been defined as the loss of skeletal muscle mass and strength that occurs with advancing age and has also been related to many metabolic diseases. In late stages, sarcopenia precedes cachexia, defined as a multifactorial syndrome characterized by an ongoing skeletal muscle wasting, with or without loss of fat mass, associated with poor prognosis in diseases, worsening quality of life and survival. Heart failure and cancer-associated cachexia represents a progressive involuntary weight loss and is mainly the result of an imbalance in the muscle protein synthesis and degradation, inflammation, and oxidative stress, causing muscle wasting. Importantly, both diseases are still the main causes of death worldwide and the molecular basis of cachexia is still poorly understood. Recently, non-coding RNAs have been described to regulate the cardiac and cancer-associated cachexia. On the other hand, exercise training is a promising ally in slowing down cachexia and improving the quality of life of patients. New studies demonstrate that exercise training, acting through non-coding RNAs, may be able to mitigate muscle wasting, as protein turnover, mitochondrial biogenesis, and antioxidant capacity improvement. This review will therefore discuss the molecular mechanisms associated with the muscle wasting in both cardiac and cancer cachexia, as well as highlighting the effects of exercise training in attenuating the loss of muscle mass in these specific conditions.

Keywords: cancer, cardiovascular diseases, exercise, muscle wasting, non-coding RNAs

1. Introduction

Cardiovascular diseases (CVD) and cancer (CA) are the two leading causes of death worldwide, representing about 28 million deaths per year [1–4]. Only CVDs affected 523 million cases worldwide, representing the main cause with 18 million deaths each year [4]. Currently, CA is the second disease in the number of deaths in the world, but its prevalence has been increasing in recent years and, in some countries, it is the main cause of death [5]. GLOBOCAN data show that in 2021,

19.3 million new cases and 10 million deaths from the CA disease were reported [6]. Considering the worldwide increase in the prevalence of CA and the high mortality from CVD, both diseases represent a serious public health problem.

The heart failure (HF) is the final common pathway of most cardiac and circulatory diseases [7]. The American Heart Association (AHA) defined HF as clinical syndrome characterized by typical symptoms such as edema, dyspnea, and fatigue; caused by changes in cardiac function and structure, with reduced cardiac contraction and/or increased intraventricular pressure at rest and physical stress [7–9]. In addition to central cardiac alterations, HF promotes changes in peripheral structure and function, impairing oxidative metabolism accompanied by microvascular rarefaction and skeletal muscle wasting [8, 10–12]. These changes in skeletal muscles contribute to reduced quality of life and increased mortality. Worldwide, HF affects more than 23 million people [7, 9], and just in the United States, around 6 million American citizens are affected, leading to more than 1 million hospitalizations/year and a mortality rate of 1 in every 9 patients hospitalized [2]. Furthermore, worsen projections are expected for the next 10 years, with an increase of 46% in cases, generating an estimated annual expenditure of 70 billion dollars, making a health epidemic [2, 13, 14].

In CA, studies have been shown that is a group of diseases characterized by uncontrolled cell growth, spreading and progressing to other cells beyond physiological limits, affecting any organ and tissue in the human body [1]. In 2021, 2.2 million new cases of breast CA have been reported worldwide, thus being the most prevalent, followed by lung CA (2.1 million), colon and rectum (1.8 million), and prostate (1.3 million). Regarding mortality, lung CA is the most lethal in the world followed by breast CA [15, 16].

Even with new drugs and therapies, there is still an increase in the prevalence of both diseases [6, 17]. Furthermore, the progression of HF and CA is related to muscle wasting and loss of body weight as well as consequent weakness toward to important clinical consequences in these diseases [18, 19]. Numerous studies demonstrate that involuntary body weight reduction, with increased muscle wasting, is the main sign of cachexia, represented by a multifactorial syndrome related to pre-established chronic diseases [18, 20]. Currently, in the world, 12 million patients have cachexia, which is responsible for worsting prognoses on established diseases, reduced quality of life, impaired therapeutic effectiveness, and increased mortality [21, 22].

To date, there are no effective pharmacological treatments for cachexia for both HF and CA [17, 23]. On the other hand, exercise training (ET) is a non-pharmacological treatment, relatively cheap and safe. In addition, ET promotes anabolic stimuli, which may preserve the muscle wasting, and at the same time enhance the quality of life and reduce mortality in cachexia patient [18, 24, 25]. During the last decades, the class of non-coding RNAs (ncRNAs): microRNAs (miRNAs), long non-coding RNAs (lncRNAs), and circular RNAs (circRNAs) have been demonstrating important associations with CVD, CA [26, 27], and with the muscle wasting promoted by cachexia [28, 29], becoming a promising mechanism to the understanding cardiac and CA cachexia.

Although great advances have been made to understand HF and CA, the mechanisms involved in skeletal muscle abnormalities, still poorly understood [3, 12, 15, 30, 31]. Therefore, understanding the mechanisms and pathways involved in skeletal muscle structure and function may help to develop new therapeutic strategies against cachexia, resulting in improved treatment and quality of life for patients [20, 32]. Consequently, this review aims to discuss the molecular mechanisms, involving ncRNAs in cardiac and CA cachexia. In addition, to known the implication of ET and ncRNAs in the treatment of cachexia.

2. Cachexia in heart failure and cancer

Cachexia (from the Greek 'kakos' for bad, and 'hexis' for condition) was first described, as a result of chronic disease, in 1860 by the French physician Charles Mauriac, which consider only as muscle disease, close to a metabolic syndrome [25, 33, 34]. Over the years, the term cachexia has been updated and nowadays is considered as a multifactorial syndrome characterized by loss of appetite, body weight (with significant muscle wasting), which may or not extend to adipose tissue. The advancement of cachexia decreases muscle function, worse fatigue, and reduces the quality of life and life expectancy of patients [21, 25, 35]. Also, recent studies demonstrate that cachexia can communicate with multiple organs, such as the heart, adipose tissue, intestine, kidneys, and liver, helping the development and progression of disease [31, 36].

Among the chronic diseases that commonly progress to cachexia, HF and CA have the largest number of affected patients [37]. Anker et al. [38] were the first authors to describe muscle wasting in HF patients, where patients with reduced body weight were diagnosed with cardiac cachexia. In 2012, the European Society of Cardiology (ESC) recognized cachexia as a comorbidity of HF [39] and in 2016 the ESC began to recommend the non-reduction of body weight in HF for obese or overweight patients [40]. In HF, the involuntary loss of body weight is considered an independent factor to reduce physical capacity, and poorer quality of life [38, 41].

The cardiac cachexia prognosis is extremely complex, with annual mortality about 20 to 40%, reaching up to 50% of patients death after 18 months of diagnosis [37, 38]. On the other hand, the cardiac cachexia incidence can range from 10–39%, depending on study design and HF patients prognosis [42, 43]. In the SICA-HF study (studies investigating co-morbidities aggravating HF), investigated cardiac caquexia in 207 HF patients with reduced ejection fraction (HFrEF) and preserved (HFpEF), of these 21% had cachexia independent of ejection fraction [44]. Studies show that cardiac cachexia would be more present in patients with HFrEF, being associated with a 3-fold higher risk of death from all causes compared to those with HFpEF [38]. On the other hand, implications of cardiac cachexia in patients with HFpEF still need further studies [42]. Valentova et al. [42], based on their clinical experience, reported that patients with HFpEF shows cardiac cachexia signs only in advanced stages of HF, possibly acting in a different biological pathway in the development of the disease [45].

Numerous changes between central and peripheral organs were observed in patients with HF [46], followed by abnormalities in skeletal muscle such as capillary rarefaction, type I to II fiber switch, impaired oxidative metabolism, decreased excitation-contraction coupling, and muscle atrophy [47, 48]. In general, cardiac cachexia is responsible for muscle atrophy in the early stages of the disease and may progress to loss of adipose tissue, just in the late stages of the disease [42]. Regarding myocardial impairment in cardiac cachexia, more solid data are needed to help distinguish the structural and functional changes related to cardiac disease from those found in cardiac cachexia. Currently, contradictory data demonstrate cardiomyocytes wasting with or without cardiac impairment [22, 49]. It is necessary to emphasize to achieve correct values of cardiac cachexia it is necessary to exclude edema values from the total body weight, a difficult task for patients with HF that hinders the accurate diagnosis of cardiac cachexia [32].

In CA, depending on the stage and development of the disease, 80% of patients have cachexia, leading to death of 30% of these patients [15, 50]. Fearon et al. [51] classifies CA cachexia into 3 stages: pre-cachexia, cachexia, and refractory cachexia. It is necessary to understand that not all patients will go through the

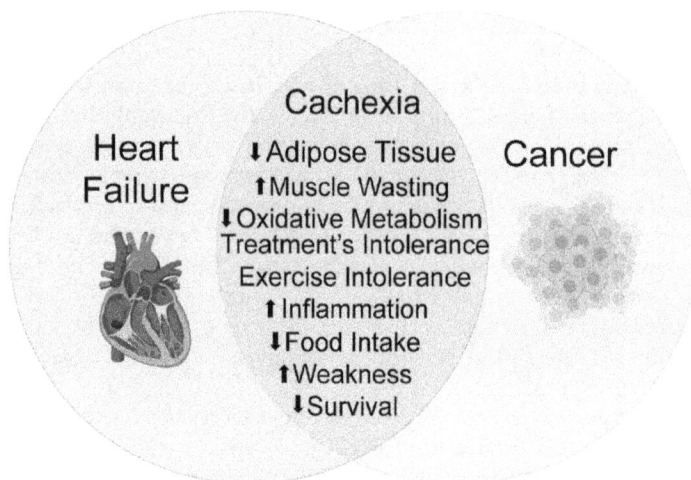

Figure 1.
Common symptoms of cardiac and cancer cachexia.

three stages. Then, the type and stage of CA can influence the progression of cachexia, as well as systemic inflammation, low food intake. In addition, CA cachexia can reduce tolerance to responses to chemotherapy treatments, worsening the prognosis of patients [50, 52].

Regarding the incidence of CA cachexia, the type of cancer may influence, since patients with gastric or pancreatic CA have over 80% of incidence. On the other hand, patients with lung, prostate, or colon CA have an incidence of 50%, and 40% of patients with advanced breast, head, and neck tumors and some leukemias develop the syndrome [35, 53, 54].

Both cardiac and CA cachexia share symptoms, as described in **Figure 1**, but cardiac cachexia presents a slower and more gradual muscle wasting [55] when compared to CA, with a progressive and rapid muscle wasting, leading to earlier death compared to cachexia from cardiac causes [56]. The international consensus for the diagnosis of cachexia is similar between HF and AC, namely: body weight loss >5% or > 2% in individuals with low BMI (< 20 kg/m^2) or loss of skeletal muscle mass in 12 months [31, 51].

3. Non-coding RNAs in cardiac and cancer cachexia

Several factors are involved to cardiac and CA cachexia like imbalance between protein synthesis and degradation, high inflammatory levels, and metabolic dysfunction (**Figure 2**). However, the pathophysiological mechanisms involved in muscle wasting induced by cardiac and CA cachexia are not fully understood. Thus, in recent years, researchers have been identifying a set of ncRNAs, with great regulatory potential in skeletal muscle, and that may have important roles in controlling muscle wasting in cachexia [29, 57].

ncRNAs are RNA molecules not translated into proteins, organized in classes depending on their structure. miRNAs have approximately 19–25 nucleotides (nt) and play a regulatory function in gene expression, through translation inhibition of messenger RNA (mRNA). The lncRNAs have approximately 200 nt in their composition and primarily interact with mRNA, DNA, protein, and miRNA and consequently regulate gene expression at the epigenetic, transcriptional,

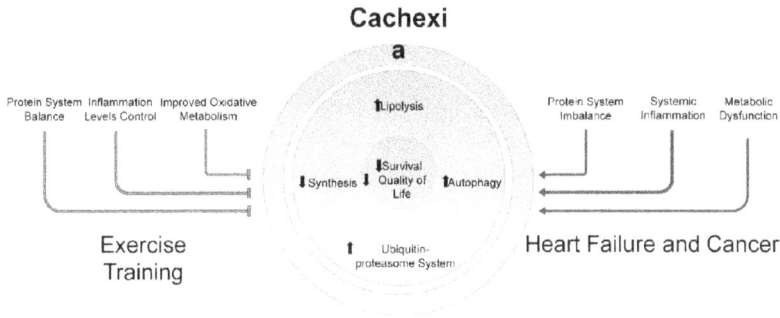

Figure 2.
Factors contributing to cardiac and cancer cachexia and the role of exercise in reversing these damages.

post-transcriptional, translational, and post-translational levels in a variety of ways. CircRNAs is produced by the circularization of specific exons by covalently linking the 3′ end of one exon to the 5′ end of another. It is known to function as a kind of miRNA sponge, thus regulating transcription, splicing, and production of peptides by translation [58, 59].

Among the ncRNAs, miRNAs have been the most studied to date due to be essential to numerous cellular functions, from fetal formation to disease development [59, 60]. miRNAs are expressed in all body tissues, but in skeletal muscle, 25% of all expressed are muscle-specific, and play important roles on muscle mass and homeostasis [29, 61]. These muscle-specific miRNAs are termed "myomiRs", and include miRNA-1, −133a, −133b, −206, −208a, −208b, −486, and − 499. Because myomiRs are exclusively expressed or enriched in striated muscle (skeletal muscle and cardiac), they occupy essential functions in the regulatory networks of myogenesis, fiber type composition, muscle growth, and metabolism [60–64]. Beyond the myomiRs, some miRNAs (e.g., miRNA-21, −24, −29b, −199, −214) shows important roles in atrophy, especially in cachexia, and known as "atromiRs" [57, 63].

Both lncRNAs and circRNAs shows important regulation on skeletal muscle and diseases such as HF and CA [29, 59, 65, 66]. Professor Chen's group, in recent years, has been investigating the lncRNAs on the molecular mechanisms of skeletal muscle mass development and control. In their works, it was found more than 4,400 lncRNAs related to atrophy mechanisms in C2C12 cells (i.e., myoblasts) [67, 68]. In the same way, circRNAs have also been related to the development and control of skeletal muscle mass [65, 68]. Although ncRNAs have a promising future, further research is needed to better understand the ncRNAs on muscle wasting mechanisms in cardiac and CA cachexia. Thus, the next topics presents the new perspectives of ncRNAs in cardiac and CA cachexia.

3.1 Cardiac cachexia and non-coding RNAs

Currently, ncRNAs are associated with molecular mechanisms in HF, responsible for progression, treatment, and use as biomarkers of the disease [59, 69, 70]. On the other hand, studies involving muscle wasting, ncRNAs, and HF remain rare. Moraes et al. [71] was the first group to investigate cardiac cachexia and ncRNAs. The study identified several changes in the regulatory pathways, such as cellular matrix, protein degradation, metabolism, c-Jun N-terminal kinase (JNK) cascade, and cellular response to the transforming growth factor-beta (TGF-β) in soleus muscle from cardiac cachexia animal. Indeed, the cellular responses found are close to those have found in patients with cardiac cachexia [24]. Furthermore, the authors demonstrated 18 differentially expressed miRNAs, where 5 was down-regulated (miRNA-30d, −146b, −214, −489 and − 632) and 13 was up-regulated (miRNA-27a, −29a, −29b, − 132, −136, −204, −210, −322, 331, −337, −376c, −434 and − 539). After gene ontology analysis, all miRNAs showed enriched to the muscle mass control pathway (**Figure 3**) [71]. However, most of the reported miRNAs were different from those usually found in skeletal muscle atrophies (e.i., induced by other etiologies, such as dystrophies, diabetes, and denervation) [72, 73], but they were close to those altered in HF and cardiac remodeling [71]; suggesting a unique profile of miRNAs responsible for muscle wasting in cardiac cachexia.

In HF, most miRNAs were found differentially expressed in both heart and skeletal muscle [63]. Moreover, many of these miRNAs are also found in blood circulation, probably allowing myocardium-skeletal muscle cross-talking, through miRNAs circulating between tissues. This communication is not exclusive to miRNAs, but it is common to all ncRNAs through lipid vesicles or proteins (e.g., exosomes) [59]. In fact, cell culture experiments have already shown that distinct cells such as cardiac fibroblasts, endothelial cells, cardiomyocytes, myoblasts, and myotubes can communicate with each other through exosomes-miRNAs [74, 75]. Therefore, during cardiac cachexia, muscle wasting probably is influenced by other tissues, such as the myocardium, through miRNAs leading to molecular changes in cachexia development [63]. In conclusion, myocardium-skeletal muscle communication via miRNAs still needs better investigation, but it sets a great precedent to understand the role of miRNAs in HF-derived dysfunctions and cardiac cachexia.

Although lncRNAs and circRNAs are not fully understood in the context of cardiac cachexia, preliminary studies have been shown a regulatory potential in the development of HF [59, 66], and skeletal muscle regulation [29, 65].

As seen above, muscle wasting in cardiac cachexia patients is an important limiting factor in daily activities and quality of life [25]. Muscle wasting is a consequence of imbalance of synthesis, and degradation protein [76]. In the last years, cardiac cachexia studies have focused on the ubiquitin-proteasome (UPP) and autophagy/lysosomal proteolytic pathways to understand the muscle wasting process [57, 77–79]. The UPP plays an important role in the breakdown of myofibrillar proteins in cardiac cachexia [80]. Proteolytic activity, through the UPP, depends on the limited expression of enzymes, which include the E3 ubiquitin-ligases muscle RING finger 1 (MurRF1) and muscle atrophy F-box (atrogin-1). The expression of these enzymes is determined by transcription factors such as the forkhead box O (FOXO) family [25, 57]. The increased expression of miRNA-18a

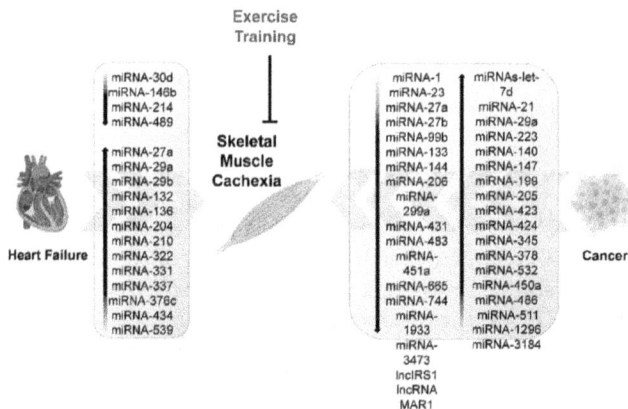

Figure 3.
Non-coding RNAs involved in cardiac and cancer cachexia.

up-regulate atrogin-1 and MuRF-1 expression; otherwise, reduced expression of miRNA-18a down-regulates FOXO3 expression, controlling myotube hypertrophy [81]. miRNA-29 plays a central role in cachexia, affecting protein synthesis and degradation pathways [57]. The increased expression of miRNA-29b led to muscle wasting with high expression of MuRF-1 and atrogin-1 and genes involved in autophagy [57]. The miRNA-23a antagomiR administration, an oligonucleotide, which acts as a competitive inhibitor of miRNA-23a, increased the expression of MuRF-1, revealing itself as an important negative regulator of the UPP [82].

The lncRNA HOX Transcript Antisense RNA (HOTAIR) can assume epigenetic functions, binding to E3 ubiquitin-ligases facilitating protein degradation through the UPP [83]. Also, the lncRNA cardiac hypertrophy-associated transcript (Chest) may regulate autophagy helping cardiomyocyte hypertrophy, and its expression was found to be increased in cardiac disease patients [84]. CircNfix is a key circRNA in cardiac muscle regeneration and regulation, whereas reducing circNfix expression promotes cell proliferation, angiogenesis, and reduced cell death [85]. CircNfix promotes the interaction of Ybx1, a transcription factor related to cell proliferation, and Nedd41, an E3 ubiquitin-ligases. Additionally, circNfix acts as a miRNA-214 sponge to promote glycogen synthase 3-β (GSK-3β) expression, a protein synthesis pathway inhibitor [85].

Protein synthesis is also essential to maintain skeletal muscle during HF [76, 86, 87]. The stimulation of phosphoinositide 3-kinase-serine/serine–threonine protein kinase (PI3K/Akt) pathway is stimulated by the insulin-like growth factor 1 (IGF-1), leading to an increase in activation of mammalian target of rapamycin (mTOR) [88]. The IGF-1/PI3K/Akt/mTOR pathway is the major signaling pathway known in skeletal muscle protein synthesis control [89, 90]. Indeed, mTOR activation-induced protein synthesis, allowing complex signals, such as TORC1 activating the ribosomal protein S6 kinase (p70S6k) and eukaryotic translation initiation factor 4E-Binding protein 1 (4E-BP1) pathways and TORC2 controlling the autophagy process [79, 91]. In cardiac cachexia, IGF-1 is down-regulated, promoting lower protein synthesis and increased degradation, aiding in muscle wasting [25].

The myomiRs-1 and -133a participate in several roles in cell development, differentiation, and growth. Besides, both have been validated to target IGF-1 [92–94], and reduction in both expression induces skeletal muscle hypertrophy [74, 95, 96]. On the other hand, increased expression of miRNA-1 and -133a can lead to muscle atrophy [63]. The binding of IGF-1 to its receptor, insulin receptor substrate 1 (IRS-1), active, through its own phosphorylation, the PI3K/AKT/mTOR signaling pathway [25]. In this way, miRNA-378 performs an important anti-hypertrophic role, acting as an inhibitor of IRS-1 via AMP-activated protein kinase (AMPK) signaling [97]. Furthermore, the miRNA-1 low expression in HF muscle patients reduce the protein expression of phosphatase and tensin homolog (PTEN), an important protein in the regulation of the synthesis pathway [98]. Bioinformatics analyzes demonstrated that miRNA-22 expression target PTEN and Sirtuin 1 protein, both responsible to regulate hypertrophy in cardiomyocytes [99, 100]. On the other hand, the synthesis pathway inhibits the FOXO family and GSK-3β leading to increased protein synthesis [25]. In HF animal models, the increase in miRNA-29 expression regulates the function of GSK-3 β, preventing hypertrophy via the nuclear factor of activated T cell (NFAT) [101]. Likewise, the miRNA-29 down-regulation leads to muscle atrophy in C2C12 cells and in cardiac cachexia patients [71]. The miRNA-23a, −132 and − 212 are related to the suppression of FOXO3, the main isoform of the FOXO family, responsible for the regulation of protein synthesis [102, 103].

Although the CircRNA SLC8A1–1 (circSLC8A1–1) has not been observed in HF yet, the circRNA expression is directly related to hypertrophy, acting as a sponge for miRNA-133 [94]. Another circRNA identified as HRCR was the first circRNA related to cardiac hypertrophy, and it is down-regulated in cardiac hypertrophy animal models, while miRNA-223 expression was increased. HRCR acts as a sponge for miRNA-223 controlling hypertrophy [104]. The muscle wasting mechanisms in cardiac cachexia are complex, and not fully understood. At the moment, ncRNAs seem to be indispensable. However, ncRNAs constitute a diverse class of molecules capable act in gene expression and skeletal muscle homeostasis. In cachexia, many of these ncRNAs are differently expressed, imply functional changes, and aggravate the progression of the disease. Further studies are needed to better understand the pathophysiological mechanisms of cardiac cachexia under ncRNAs participation.

3.2 Cancer cachexia and non-coding RNAs

In silico and *in vivo* approaches demonstrated the involvement of miRNAs-21 and -206 in the regulation of muscle wasting from different atrophic models (i.e. diabetes, cancer cachexia, chronic renal failure, fasting, and denervation) by targeting the transcription factor YY1 and the translational initiator factor eIF4E3, indicating these miRNAs as fine-tuning regulators from muscle catabolism [73]. The tumor-secreted miRNA-21 and -29a showed an activation of premetastatic inflammatory pathways, mediated by its binding to the Toll Like Receptor (TLR), such as, murine TLR7 and human TLR8. CA-induced miRNA-21 was also found to be overexpressed in exosomes during tumor evolution, which signals through the TLR7 on myoblasts to promote cell apoptosis [105, 106].

A recent meta-analysis showed that miRNAs are related to muscle wasting during CA cachexia, including miRNAs-27a, −27b, −140 and -199a. These miRNAs favor atrophy and also inhibit muscle growth [107].

In studies using wild-type mice and poly (ADP-ribose) polymerases- 1(Parp-1) $^-/^-$ and Parp-2 $^-/^-$ with Lewis lung carcinoma revealed that the miRNA-1 was found down-regulated in the skeletal muscle of these animals. Furthermore, miRNA-133a was reduced in the diaphragm and gastrocnemius of animals with Parp-2 $^-/^-$, while animals with Parp-1 $^-/^-$ showed difference only in the reduction of the diaphragm. The expression of miRNA-206 and -486 in tumor bearing-mice was also lower in wild-type animals. There was proliferation and differentiation of muscle cells in Parp-1 $^-/^-$ mice via miRNA-133a, −206, and − 486 action, while the inhibition of Parp-2 through miRNA-206 promoted the differentiation of muscle cells in the gastrocnemius muscle [108].

Lee et al. [109] performed analysis in CA cachectic mice whereas they found 9 differentially expressed miRNAs, namely: miRNA-147, −205, −223, −299a, −431, −511, −665, −1933 and -3473d, most of all involved in many functions, such as cell growth, signaling, inflammatory response, and catabolism [109]. In another study, with CA cachexia patients, 5 miRNAs were found differently expressed. Of these, miRNA-23a, −99b, −483 and − 744 were down-regulated, and miRNA-378 was up-regulated in these patients and were involved with catecholamine-stimulated lipolysis in adipocytes [110].

Patients with CA cachexia showed up-regulation of 8 miRNAs, which were involved in myogenesis, muscle metabolism and inflammation (miRNAs-let-7d, −199a, −345, −423, −532, −1296 and − 3184) [111]. A study using vastus lateralis biopsy showed a higher expression of miRNA-424, and -450a and a lower expression of miRNA-144 and -451a. These processes involved target genes related to IL-6, TGF-β, TNFα, insulin and Akt pathway, thus contributing to a reduction in the survival of these patients [112].

Regarding lncRNAs in cachectic animals, lncIRS1 was described to act as a sponge for miRNA-15, regulating the expression of IRS1. When this lncRNA is overexpressed, it activates the signaling pathways IGF-1 / PI3K / Akt, thus increasing protein synthesis. Furthermore, this increase in its expression inhibits muscle wasting. When suppressed, there is a decrease in IGF-1 levels in favor to muscle wasting [113]. LncRNA muscle anabolic regulator 1 (MAR1) showed an interaction with miRNA-487b promoting muscle regeneration and differentiation; when overexpressed, it has been shown to attenuate muscle wasting, thus being a possible therapeutic target for CA cachexia [114]. Another lncRNA that was shown to be altered in CA cachexia was cachexia-related long noncoding RNA1 (CAAlnc1), which through its interaction with the protein Hu antigen R (HuR), an essential protein for adipogenesis, led to fat loss [115].

lncMyoD is a lncRNA activated during myoblast differentiation directly by Myogenic Differentiation 1 (MyoD). When overexpressed, it has been shown to inhibit muscle differentiation and cell cycle exit, thus being associated with CA cachexia patients [116]. Recently, the lncRNA metastasis associated lung adenocarcinoma transcript 1 (MALAT1) was found involved in expression of peroxisome proliferator activated gamma receptor (PPAR-y), at the transcriptional level, associating with fat loss, and reflect a marker of worse prognosis to affected CA cachexia patients [117].

Looking for circRNAs, only one study to date has shown the expression of circRNA Hsa_circ_0010522 (ciRNA-133) in gastric CA. These circRNA was positively associated with body fat and brown fat mass. ciRNA-133 has been shown to interact as a sponge with miRNA-133 in an *in vivo* approach. When ciRNA-133 was overexpressed in mice, it was also shown to be increased in tumors tissue. The animals showed reduced inguinal adipose tissue mass and darkening. Therefore, ciRNA-133 worsens cancer cachexia, probably through the darkening of the fat [118].

The **Figure 3** indicates the ncRNAs that have been identified to promote cardiac and cancer cachexia.

4. Non-coding RNAs and physical exercise on skeletal muscle

The health benefits of ET have been recognized for decades [119, 120]. Currently, ET is an important component in the prevention and treatment of HF and CA diseases [121, 122], as well as other chronic diseases [123]. Furthermore, being widely recommended by AHA, ESC and American Cancer Society (ACS) guidelines [124, 125]. On the other hand, no effective pharmacological therapies are available in the treatment to cachexia [20]. Indeed, ET acts directly on adaptations in skeletal muscle metabolism and morphology, inducing anabolic stimuli, which reduce muscle wasting and improve in morbidity and mortality in cachexia patient [17, 18, 24, 25, 126].

Recent studies suggest the involvement of ncRNAs, especially miRNAs, on ET-induced skeletal muscle [120, 127] and myocardium [128, 129] adaptation. In this way, potential role of ET on miRNA–mRNA networks were associated with muscle mass control, whereas ET induces skeletal muscle metabolic and myogenic pathways through miRNAs modulation [120, 130].

Although only a limited number of lncRNAs have been characterized in response to ET, the expectation of possible applications of these ncRNAs is huge. Recent study showed, through a bioinformatics analysis, the expression of lncRNAs in different ET modalities including resistance training, endurance training, high-intensity interval training, and combined ET [131]. These lncRNAs were involved with signaling pathways, such as: collagen fibril organization, extracellular matrix organization, myoblast and plasma membrane fusion, skeletal muscle contraction, synaptic transmission, PI3K/Akt/mTOR regulation, autophagy, and angiogenesis [131]. Studies validating the expression of these lncRNAs in trained human samples still needs to be evaluated. The large number of cellular functions regulated by lncRNAs and affected by ET open space for countless possibilities, becoming very promising for the future.

Even in the beginning, research involving ET and circRNAs regulation may demonstrate a possible mechanism in muscle wasting. Guo et al. [132] identified 21 circRNAs differently expressed in trained animals compared to sedentary ones. Among them, circRNA BBS9 was found reduced in aging compared to young mice and elevated expression in ET compared to sedentary aging mice. In fact, CircRNA BBS9 acts as a sponge for 10 distinct miRNAs, regulating metabolic and the PI3K/Akt/mTOR signaling pathway [132]. Besides their functions in skeletal muscle, circRNAs are promising ET biomarkers. In this way, circRNA MBOAT2 has been used in marathon athletes for cardiorespiratory assessment [133]. There are many regulatory possibilities linked to ET and ncRNAs. However, few works directly involved ncRNAs, ET, and cachexia in the literature. Below we will summarize the main findings involving this theme.

4.1 Cardiac cachexia, non-coding RNAs and physical exercise

More the one decade ago, ET was established as an important non-pharmacological strategy for HF treatment, promoting important adaptations in neurohormonal control and cardiac function [126, 134, 135]. Moreover, ET provide different biochemical, structural, and functional skeletal muscle adaptations, acting against the HF progression, and promoting capillarization, fiber type shift, oxidative metabolism improvement, and antioxidant defenses [136–138]. Important to note, skeletal muscles are highly responsive to ET stimulus [48], being able to reduce muscle wasting pathways, with E3 ligases mRNA down-regulation [77] and increasing protein synthesis (**Figure 2**) [48].

Many of miRNAs were altered in heart, circulation, and skeletal muscle after ET [139, 140]. Souza et al. [141] evaluated ET adaptations in rats with HF. The authors found 56 miRNAs differentially expressed in the trained group compared to sedentary. Of these, 38 miRNAs were up-regulated, and 18 miRNAs were down-regulated in trained rats. This miRNAs profile were involved with cell death, inflammation, cell metabolism, and morphology pathways [141]. Also, treadmill training may reduce the expression of miRNA-1 and -133 in the hearts of rats which are negative regulators in protein synthesis [142]. In contrast, swimming training increased expression of miRNA-21 and -144 targeting PTEN and miRNA-145 targeting tuberous sclerosis complex 2 (TSC2) [139]; whereas miRNA-124 targeting PI3K was down-regulated involved with ET-induced physiological ventricular hypertrophy. Furthermore, miRNA-17 was up-regulated in the bloodstream of exercised patients with HF, as well as rats, after ET. This increase is responsible to promote cardiomyocytes hypertrophy and proliferation, acting indirectly through PTEN and Akt signaling pathway [143]. miRNAs also regulate ET adaptation acutely, after accomplished a marathon miRNA-1, −133a, −206, and − 499 were abundantly expressed in the circulation, and 24 hours after all miRNAs, except miRNA-499, returned to baseline values. It shows that maybe these miRNAs were necessary to regulate protein synthesis in an acute way [144]. Besides, the same miRNAs were found differently expressed after 4 weeks of ET in the bloodstream, being involved in protein synthesis [145]. In conclusion, ET through miRNAs can induce molecular mechanisms related to muscle trophism acutely and chronically.

Compared to miRNAs, lncRNAs and circRNAs actions on exercise- induced muscle wasting protection remain unknown. In the heart, Lin et al. (2021) [129] evaluated the ET effects on lncRNAs expression induced by aortic constriction, showing a markedly increase in lncRNA Mhrt779 expression compared to sedentary ones. Mhrt779 expression inhibited cardiac remodeling through Hdac2/Akt/GSK-3β pathway [129]. Consequently, the lncRNAs studies are extremely important and will help to understand the ET and ncRNA in CVD, in both heart and skeletal muscle tissue.

4.2 Cancer cachexia, non-coding RNAs and physical exercise

The therapeutic strategy for CA cachexia is still open to a new treatment. However, physical fitness maintenance is widely recommended in the early disease stages [146–148]. ET attenuates CA cachexia effects through several mechanisms, such as anabolic increase, muscle homeostasis, improvement of insulin sensitivity, and control inflammation levels (**Figure 2**). Both aerobic ET and resistance ET were capable to reduce inflammation, through the balance of the pro and anti-inflammatory cytokines, namely TNFα, IL-6, and IL-10. In animals, this modulation, through exercise, reduced tumor volume and muscle wasting [149–151].

After resistance ET, miRNA-1 expression was down-regulated in young men and is responsible for skeletal muscle hypertrophy. In addition, miRNA-126 also induce hypertrophy by IGF-1 pathway and was down-regulated after acute exercise [131]. The PI3K/Akt/mTOR signaling pathway, once reduced either by age or disease progression, can be re-established with resistance ET [132]. ET restores the expression of 26 miRNAs differentially expressed with aging. Among these miRNAs, the family of miRNA-99 and -100, show important regulation on PI3K/Akt/mTOR signaling pathway, increasing protein synthesis, and preventing skeletal muscle atrophy [133].

Regarding muscle wasting, aerobic ET has been shown to stimulate skeletal muscle hypertrophy, reducing autophagy and the expression of E3 ubiquitin-ligases (i.e., Murf and Atrogin-1) [152, 153]. A study with the Walker-256 tumor showed that ET was able to reduce muscle wasting and to control TNF-α and IL-6 levels, oxidative damage, and E3 ubiquitin-ligases expression, acting as an anti-atrophy treatment [154]. Curiously, a study using low-intensity ET was able to inhibit the activation of the UPP and re-active mTOR pathway, suppressing phosphorylated AMPK, thus indicating that the low-intensity exercise was able to prevent CA cachexia muscle wasting [155].

Since myomiRs are tightly regulated during ET, it has been suggested that they could be used as biomarkers for monitoring cachectic patients avoiding harmful exercise, or as biomarkers for drugs that mimic exercise, such as trimetazidine [77]. In this sense, circulating miRNAs were shown to act like a biomarker for muscle loss, regeneration, therapeutic efficacy, and early detection of cachexia. We can highlight the miRNAs-130a [156], −21 [157], −203 [158], −486 [159], and myomiRs: miRNAs-1, −133a, −133b e − 206 [160–162].

5. Conclusion

Cachexia has been described as a serious health problem due to its prevalence and by affects several organs and systems. The development of cardiac and CA cachexia promotes imbalance protein system, which in turn facilitates exercise intolerance and weakness, increasingly leading to death. Therefore, understanding all the mechanisms behind this syndrome and its possible biomarkers is of great value in creating new intervention strategies.

ET has been shown to have positive results as a non-pharmacological therapy for cachexia. Its effect related to decreasing muscle degradation, inflammatory environment, fatigue, and increased survival highlights its importance within the treatment protocols for these syndromes. Current HF and CA guidelines strongly recommend regular physical exercise for stable patients to prevent and/or attenuate skeletal muscle abnormalities. Its application should incorporate the early stage of cachexia development and may be accompanied by the markers previously described. Given this, its incorporation for the treatment of cachexia only needs a focus on the syndrome. Further studies should be undertaken to explore the underlying mechanisms responsible for cardiac and CA cachexia adaptations to exercise and the regulation of ncRNAs.

Acknowledgements

The authors thank the laboratory team for their technical assistance. The researchers were supported by Sao Paulo Research Foundation (FAPESP: #2015/22814-5 and #2015/17275-8), MicroRNA Research Center (NAPmiR, University of Sao Paulo), National Council for Scientific and Technological Development (CNPq: #313479/2017-8), and Coordination for the Improvement of Higher Education Personnel (CAPES-PROEX: #88887.484856/2020-2100 and #88887.640701/2021-2100).

Conflict of interest

The authors declare no conflict of interest.

Author details

Bruno Rocha de Avila Pelozin[†], Luis Felipe Rodrigues[†],
Edilamar Menezes De Oliveira and Tiago Fernandes[*]
Laboratory of Biochemistry and Molecular Biology of the Exercise, School of Physical Education and Sport, University of Sao Paulo, São Paulo, Brazil

*Address all correspondence to: tifernandes@usp.br

† Equal contribution.

IntechOpen

References

[1] World Health Organization. Cancer 2021. https://www.who.int/news-room/fact-sheets/detail/cancer.

[2] Virani SS, Alonso A, Aparicio HJ, Benjamin EJ, Bittencourt MS, Callaway CW, et al. Heart Disease and Stroke Statistics—2021 Update. Circulation 2021;143:e254–e743. DOI:10.1161/CIR.0000000000000950.

[3] Naghavi M, Abajobir AA, Abbafati C, Abbas KM, Abd-Allah F, Abera SF, et al. Global, regional, and national age-sex specific mortality for 264 causes of death, 1980-2016: a systematic analysis for the Global Burden of Disease Study 2016. Lancet 2017;390:1151-1210. DOI:10.1016/S0140-6736(17)32152-9.

[4] Roth GA, Mensah GA, Johnson CO, Addolorato G, Ammirati E, Baddour LM, et al. Global Burden of Cardiovascular Diseases and Risk Factors, 1990-2019: Update From the GBD 2019 Study. J Am Coll Cardiol 2020;76:2982-3021. DOI:10.1016/j.jacc.2020.11.010.

[5] Dagenais GR, Leong DP, Rangarajan S, Lanas F, Lopez-Jaramillo P, Gupta R, et al. Variations in common diseases, hospital admissions, and deaths in middle-aged adults in 21 countries from five continents (PURE): a prospective cohort study. Lancet (London, England) 2020;395:785-94. DOI:10.1016/S0140-6736(19)32007-0.

[6] Sung H, Ferlay J, Siegel RL, Laversanne M, Soerjomataram I, Jemal A, et al. Global Cancer Statistics 2020: GLOBOCAN Estimates of Incidence and Mortality Worldwide for 36 Cancers in 185 Countries. CA Cancer J Clin 2021;71:209-249. DOI:10.3322/caac.21660.

[7] Florido R, Kwak L, Lazo M, Nambi V, Ahmed HM, Hegde SM, et al. Six-Year Changes in Physical Activity and the Risk of Incident Heart Failure: ARIC Study. Circulation 2018;137:2142-2151. DOI:10.1161/CIRCULATIONAHA.117.030226.

[8] Del Buono MG, Arena R, Borlaug BA, Carbone S, Canada JM, Kirkman DL, et al. Exercise Intolerance in Patients With Heart Failure. J Am Coll Cardiol 2019;73:2209-2225. DOI:10.1016/j.jacc.2019.01.072.

[9] Bozkurt B, Coats AJ, Tsutsui H, Abdelhamid M, Adamopoulos S, Albert N, et al. Universal Definition and Classification of Heart Failure. J Card Fail 2021;27:387-413. DOI:10.1016/j.cardfail.2021.01.022.

[10] Anker SD, Swank JW, Volterrani M, Chua TP, Clark AL, Poole-Wilson PA, et al. The influence of muscle mass, strength, fatigability and blood flow on exercise capacity in cachectic and non-cachectic patients with chronic heart failure. Eur Heart J 1997;18:259-269. DOI:10.1093/oxfordjournals.eurheartj.a015229.

[11] Brum PC, Bacurau A V., Cunha TF, Bechara LRG, Moreira JBN. Skeletal myopathy in heart failure: effects of aerobic exercise training. Exp Physiol 2014;99:616-620. DOI:10.1113/expphysiol.2013.076844.

[12] Kennel PJ, Mancini DM, Schulze PC. Skeletal Muscle Changes in Chronic Cardiac Disease and Failure. Compr. Physiol., vol. 5, Wiley; 2015, p. 1947-69. DOI:10.1002/cphy.c110003.

[13] Dunlay SM, Roger VL, Redfield MM. Epidemiology of heart failure with preserved ejection fraction. Nat Rev Cardiol 2017;14:591-602. DOI:10.1038/nrcardio.2017.65.

[14] Mishra S, Kass DA. Cellular and molecular pathobiology of heart failure with preserved ejection fraction. Nat

Rev Cardiol 2021;18:400-423. DOI:10.1038/s41569-020-00480-6.

[15] De Matuoka E Chiocchetti G, Lopes-Aguiar L, Da Silva Miyaguti NA, Viana LR, De Moraes Salgado C, Orvoën OO, et al. A time-course comparison of skeletal muscle metabolomic alterations in walker-256 tumour-bearing rats at different stages of life. Metabolites 2021;11. DOI:10.3390/metabo11060404.

[16] Siegel RL, Miller KD, Jemal A. Cancer statistics, 2020. CA Cancer J Clin 2020;70:7-30. DOI:10.3322/caac.21590.

[17] Lena A, Anker MS, Springer J. Muscle Wasting and Sarcopenia in Heart Failure-The Current State of Science. Int J Mol Sci 2020;21. DOI:10.3390/ijms21186549.

[18] von Haehling S. The wasting continuum in heart failure: from sarcopenia to cachexia. Proc Nutr Soc 2015;74:367-377. DOI:10.1017/S0029665115002438.

[19] Argilés JM, Busquets S, Stemmler B, López-Soriano FJ. Cancer cachexia: understanding the molecular basis. Nat Rev Cancer 2014;14:754-762. DOI:10.1038/nrc3829.

[20] Ebner N, Anker SD, von Haehling S. Recent developments in the field of cachexia, sarcopenia, and muscle wasting: highlights from the 12th Cachexia Conference. J Cachexia Sarcopenia Muscle 2020;11:274-285. DOI:10.1002/jcsm.12552.

[21] Roeland EJ, Bohlke K, Baracos VE, Bruera E, del Fabbro E, Dixon S, et al. Management of Cancer Cachexia: ASCO Guideline. J Clin Oncol 2020;38:2438-2453. DOI:10.1200/JCO.20.00611.

[22] Curcio F, Testa G, Liguori I, Papillo M, Flocco V, Panicara V, et al. Sarcopenia and Heart Failure. Nutrients 2020;12:211. DOI:10.3390/nu12010211.

[23] Cohen S, Nathan JA, Goldberg AL. Muscle wasting in disease: molecular mechanisms and promising therapies. Nat Rev Drug Discov 2015;14:58-74. DOI:10.1038/nrd4467.

[24] Ebner N, Elsner S, Springer J, von Haehling S. Molecular mechanisms and treatment targets of muscle wasting and cachexia in heart failure: an overview. Curr Opin Support Palliat Care 2014;8:15-24. DOI:10.1097/SPC.0000000000000030.

[25] von Haehling S, Ebner N, Dos Santos MR, Springer J, Anker SD. Muscle wasting and cachexia in heart failure: mechanisms and therapies. Nat Rev Cardiol 2017;14:323-341. DOI:10.1038/nrcardio.2017.51.

[26] Zhou B, Yang H, Yang C, Bao Y-L, Yang S-M, Liu J, et al. Translation of noncoding RNAs and cancer. Cancer Lett 2021;497:89-99. DOI:10.1016/j.canlet.2020.10.002.

[27] Li M, Duan L, Li Y, Liu B. Long noncoding RNA/circular noncoding RNA-miRNA-mRNA axes in cardiovascular diseases. Life Sci 2019;233:116440. DOI:10.1016/j.lfs.2019.04.066.

[28] Bei Y, Xiao J. MicroRNAs in muscle wasting and cachexia induced by heart failure. Nat Rev Cardiol 2017;14:566. DOI:10.1038/nrcardio.2017.122.

[29] Chen R, Lei S, Jiang T, She Y, Shi H. Regulation of Skeletal Muscle Atrophy in Cachexia by MicroRNAs and Long Non-coding RNAs. Front Cell Dev Biol 2020;8:577010. DOI:10.3389/fcell.2020.577010.

[30] Liu X, Platt C, Rosenzweig A. The Role of MicroRNAs in the Cardiac Response to Exercise. Cold Spring Harb Perspect Med 2017;7:a029850. DOI:10.1101/cshperspect.a029850.

[31] Argilés JM, Stemmler B, López-Soriano FJ, Busquets S.

Inter-tissue communication in cancer cachexia. Nat Rev Endocrinol 2018;15:9-20. DOI:10.1038/s41574-018-0123-0.

[32] Ebner N, von Haehling S. Highlights from the 9th Cachexia Conference. J Cachexia Sarcopenia Muscle 2017;8:508-511. DOI:10.1002/jcsm.12217.

[33] Doehner W, Anker SD. Cardiac cachexia in early literature: a review of research prior to Medline. Int J Cardiol 2002;85:7-14. DOI:10.1016/S0167-5273(02)00230-9.

[34] Theologides A. Pathogenesis of cachexia in cancer. A review and a hypothesis. Cancer 1972;29:484-488. DOI:10.1002/1097-0142(197202)29:2<484::AID-CNCR2820290238>3.0.CO;2-E.

[35] Peixoto da Silva S, Santos JMO, Costa e Silva MP, Gil da Costa RM, Medeiros *R. Cancer* cachexia and its pathophysiology: links with sarcopenia, anorexia and asthenia. J Cachexia Sarcopenia Muscle 2020;11:619-635. DOI:10.1002/jcsm.12528.

[36] Argilés JM, Busquets S, Stemmler B, López-Soriano FJ. Cancer cachexia: understanding the molecular basis. Nat Rev Cancer 2014;14:754-762. DOI:10.1038/nrc3829.

[37] von Haehling S, Anker MS, Anker SD. Prevalence and clinical impact of cachexia in chronic illness in Europe, USA, and Japan: facts and numbers update 2016. J Cachexia Sarcopenia Muscle 2016;7:507-509. DOI:10.1002/jcsm.12167.

[38] Anker SD, Ponikowski P, Varney S, Chua TP, Clark AL, Webb-Peploe KM, et al. Wasting as independent risk factor for mortality in chronic heart failure. Lancet (London, England) 1997;349:1050-3. DOI:10.1016/S0140-6736(96)07015-8.

[39] McMurray JJ V, Adamopoulos S, Anker SD, Auricchio A, Böhm M, Dickstein K, et al. ESC Guidelines for the diagnosis and treatment of acute and chronic heart failure 2012: The Task Force for the Diagnosis and Treatment of Acute and Chronic Heart Failure 2012 of the European Society of Cardiology. Developed in collaboration with the Heart. Eur Heart J 2012;33:1787-1847. DOI:10.1093/eurheartj/ehs104.

[40] Ponikowski P, Voors AA, Anker SD, Bueno H, Cleland JGF, Coats AJS, et al. 2016 ESC Guidelines for the diagnosis and treatment of acute and chronic heart failure: The Task Force for the diagnosis and treatment of acute and chronic heart failure of the European Society of Cardiology (ESC) Developed with the special contribution of. Eur Heart J 2016;37:2129-2200. DOI:10.1093/eurheartj/ehw128.

[41] Fülster S, Tacke M, Sandek A, Ebner N, Tschöpe C, Doehner W, et al. Muscle wasting in patients with chronic heart failure: results from the studies investigating co-morbidities aggravating heart failure (SICA-HF). Eur Heart J 2013;34:512-519. DOI:10.1093/eurheartj/ehs381.

[42] Valentova M, Anker SD, von Haehling S. Cardiac Cachexia Revisited: The Role of Wasting in Heart Failure. Heart Fail Clin 2020;16:61-69. DOI:10.1016/j.hfc.2019.08.006.

[43] Christensen HM, Kistorp C, Schou M, Keller N, Zerahn B, Frystyk J, et al. Prevalence of cachexia in chronic heart failure and characteristics of body composition and metabolic status. Endocrine 2013;43:626-634. DOI:10.1007/s12020-012-9836-3.

[44] Emami A, Saitoh M, Valentova M, Sandek A, Evertz R, Ebner N, et al. Comparison of sarcopenia and cachexia in men with chronic heart failure: results from the Studies Investigating Co-morbidities Aggravating Heart Failure (SICA-HF). Eur J Heart Fail 2018;20:1580-1587. DOI:10.1002/ejhf.1304.

[45] Tromp J, Westenbrink BD, Ouwerkerk W, van Veldhuisen DJ, Samani NJ, Ponikowski P, et al. Identifying Pathophysiological Mechanisms in Heart Failure With Reduced Versus Preserved Ejection Fraction. J Am Coll Cardiol 2018;72: 1081-1090. DOI:10.1016/j.jacc.2018. 06.050.

[46] Conraads VM, Van Craenenbroeck EM, De Maeyer C, Van Berendoncks AM, Beckers PJ, Vrints CJ. Unraveling new mechanisms of exercise intolerance in chronic heart failure: role of exercise training. Heart Fail Rev 2013;18:65-77. DOI:10.1007/ s10741-012-9324-0.

[47] Drexler H, Riede U, Münzel T, König H, Funke E, Just H. Alterations of skeletal muscle in chronic heart failure. Circulation 1992;85:1751-1759. DOI:10.1161/01.cir.85.5.1751.

[48] Alves CRR, da Cunha TF, da Paixão NA, Brum PC. Aerobic exercise training as therapy for cardiac and cancer cachexia. Life Sci 2015;125:9-14. DOI:10.1016/j.lfs.2014.11.029.

[49] Florea VG, Moon J, Pennell DJ, Doehner W, Coats AJS, Anker SD. Wasting of the left ventricle in patients with cardiac cachexia: a cardiovascular magnetic resonance study. Int J Cardiol 2004;97:15-20. DOI:10.1016/j.ijcard. 2003.05.050.

[50] Sartori R, Hagg A, Zampieri S, Armani A, Winbanks CE, Viana LR, et al. Perturbed BMP signaling and denervation promote muscle wasting in cancer cachexia. Sci Transl Med 2021;In press.

[51] Fearon K, Strasser F, Anker SD, Bosaeus I, Bruera E, Fainsinger RL, et al. Definition and classification of cancer cachexia: an international consensus. Lancet Oncol 2011;12:489-495. DOI:10.1016/S1470-2045(10)70218-7.

[52] von Haehling S, Anker SD. Cachexia as a major underestimated and unmet medical need: facts and numbers. J Cachexia Sarcopenia Muscle 2010;1:1-5. DOI:10.1007/s13539-010-0002-6.

[53] Kwon M, Kim RB, Roh J-L, Lee S-W, Kim S-B, Choi S-H, et al. Prevalence and clinical significance of cancer cachexia based on time from treatment in advanced-stage head and neck squamous cell carcinoma. Head Neck 2017;39:716-723. DOI:10.1002/ hed.24672.

[54] Jager-Wittenaar H, Dijkstra PU, Dijkstra G, Bijzet J, Langendijk JA, van der Laan BFAM, et al. High prevalence of cachexia in newly diagnosed head and neck cancer patients: An exploratory study. Nutrition 2017;35:114-118. DOI:10.1016/j. nut.2016.11.008.

[55] von Haehling S, Steinbeck L, Doehner W, Springer J, Anker SD. Muscle wasting in heart failure: An overview. Int J Biochem Cell Biol 2013;45:2257-2265. DOI:10.1016/j. biocel.2013.04.025.

[56] Fearon K, Strasser F, Anker SD, Bosaeus I, Bruera E, Fainsinger RL, et al. Definition and classification of cancer cachexia: an international consensus. Lancet Oncol 2011;12:489-495. DOI:10.1016/S1470-2045(10)70218-7.

[57] van de Worp WRPH, Theys J, van Helvoort A, Langen RCJ. Regulation of muscle atrophy by microRNAs: "AtromiRs" as potential target in cachexia. Curr Opin Clin Nutr Metab Care 2018;21:423-429. DOI:10.1097/ MCO.0000000000000503.

[58] Du G, Zhang Y, Hu S, Zhou X, Li Y. Non-coding RNAs in exosomes and adipocytes cause fat loss during cancer cachexia. Non-Coding RNA Res 2021;6:80-85. DOI:10.1016/j. ncrna.2021.04.001.

[59] Gomes CPC, Schroen B, Kuster GM, Robinson EL, Ford K, Squire IB, et al. Regulatory RNAs in Heart Failure. Circulation 2020;141:313-328. DOI:10.1161/CIRCULATIONAHA.119.042474.

[60] van Rooij E, Liu N, Olson EN. MicroRNAs flex their muscles. Trends Genet 2008;24:159-166. DOI:10.1016/j.tig.2008.01.007.

[61] Horak M, Novak J, Bienertova-Vasku J. Muscle-specific microRNAs in skeletal muscle development. Dev Biol 2016;410:1-13. DOI:10.1016/j.ydbio.2015.12.013.

[62] McCarthy JJ. MicroRNA-206: the skeletal muscle-specific myomiR. Biochim Biophys Acta 2008;1779:682-691. DOI:10.1016/j.bbagrm.2008.03.001.

[63] Murach KA, McCarthy JJ. MicroRNAs, heart failure, and aging: potential interactions with skeletal muscle. Heart Fail Rev 2017;22:209-218. DOI:10.1007/s10741-016-9572-5.

[64] van Rooij E, Quiat D, Johnson BA, Sutherland LB, Qi X, Richardson JA, et al. A family of microRNAs encoded by myosin genes governs myosin expression and muscle performance. Dev Cell 2009;17:662-673. DOI:10.1016/j.devcel.2009.10.013.

[65] Zhang P, Chao Z, Zhang R, Ding R, Wang Y, Wu W, et al. Circular RNA Regulation of Myogenesis. Cells 2019;8. DOI:10.3390/cells8080885.

[66] Wang Y, Liu B. Circular RNA in Diseased Heart. Cells 2020;9. DOI:10.3390/cells9051240.

[67] Chen R, Jiang T, She Y, Xie S, Zhou S, Li C, et al. Comprehensive analysis of lncRNAs and mRNAs with associated co-expression and ceRNA networks in C2C12 myoblasts and myotubes. Gene 2018;647:164-173. DOI:10.1016/j.gene.2018.01.039.

[68] Chen R, Lei S, Jiang T, Zeng J, Zhou S, She Y. Roles of lncRNAs and circRNAs in regulating skeletal muscle development. Acta Physiol (Oxf) 2020;228:e13356. DOI:10.1111/apha.13356.

[69] Melman YF, Shah R, Das S. MicroRNAs in heart failure: is the picture becoming less miRky? Circ Heart Fail 2014;7:203-214. DOI:10.1161/CIRCHEARTFAILURE.113.000266.

[70] Vegter EL, van der Meer P, de Windt LJ, Pinto YM, Voors AA. MicroRNAs in heart failure: from biomarker to target for therapy. Eur J Heart Fail 2016;18:457-468. DOI:10.1002/ejhf.495.

[71] Moraes LN, Fernandez GJ, Vechetti-Júnior IJ, Freire PP, Souza RWA, Villacis RAR, et al. Integration of miRNA and mRNA expression profiles reveals microRNA-regulated networks during muscle wasting in cardiac cachexia. Sci Rep 2017;7:6998. DOI:10.1038/s41598-017-07236-2.

[72] Eisenberg I, Eran A, Nishino I, Moggio M, Lamperti C, Amato AA, et al. Distinctive patterns of microRNA expression in primary muscular disorders. Proc Natl Acad Sci U S A 2007;104:17016-17021. DOI:10.1073/pnas.0708115104.

[73] Soares RJ, Cagnin S, Chemello F, Silvestrin M, Musaro A, De Pitta C, et al. Involvement of microRNAs in the regulation of muscle wasting during catabolic conditions. J Biol Chem 2014;289:21909-21925. DOI:10.1074/jbc.M114.561845.

[74] McCarthy JJ, Esser KA. MicroRNA-1 and microRNA-133a expression are decreased during skeletal muscle hypertrophy. J Appl Physiol 2007;102:306-313. DOI:10.1152/japplphysiol.00932.2006.

[75] McCarthy JJ, Esser KA, Peterson CA, Dupont-Versteegden EE. Evidence of MyomiR network regulation of beta-myosin heavy chain gene expression during skeletal muscle atrophy. Physiol Genomics 2009;39:219-226. DOI:10.1152/physiolgenomics.00042.2009.

[76] Glass DJ. Signalling pathways that mediate skeletal muscle hypertrophy and atrophy. Nat Cell Biol 2003;5:87-90. DOI:10.1038/ncb0203-87.

[77] Cunha TF, Bacurau AVN, Moreira JBN, Paixão NA, Campos JC, Ferreira JCB, et al. Exercise training prevents oxidative stress and ubiquitin-proteasome system overactivity and reverse skeletal muscle atrophy in heart failure. PLoS One 2012;7:e41701. DOI:10.1371/journal.pone.0041701.

[78] Jannig PR, Moreira JBN, Bechara LRG, Bozi LHM, Bacurau A V, Monteiro AWA, et al. Autophagy signaling in skeletal muscle of infarcted rats. PLoS One 2014;9:e85820. DOI:10.1371/journal.pone.0085820.

[79] Schiaffino S, Dyar KA, Ciciliot S, Blaauw B, Sandri M. Mechanisms regulating skeletal muscle growth and atrophy. FEBS J 2013;280:4294-4314. DOI:10.1111/febs.12253.

[80] Tisdale MJ. The ubiquitin-proteasome pathway as a therapeutic target for muscle wasting. J Support Oncol 2005;3:209-217.

[81] Liu C, Wang M, Chen M, Zhang K, Gu L, Li Q, et al. miR-18a induces myotubes atrophy by down-regulating IgfI. Int J Biochem Cell Biol 2017;90:145-154. DOI:10.1016/j.biocel.2017.07.020.

[82] Lin Z, Murtaza I, Wang K, Jiao J, Gao J, Li P-F. miR-23a functions downstream of NFATc3 to regulate cardiac hypertrophy. Proc Natl Acad Sci U S A 2009;106:12103-12108. DOI:10.1073/pnas.0811371106.

[83] Yoon J-H, Abdelmohsen K, Kim J, Yang X, Martindale JL, Tominaga-Yamanaka K, et al. Scaffold function of long non-coding RNA HOTAIR in protein ubiquitination. Nat Commun 2013;4:2939. DOI:10.1038/ncomms3939.

[84] Viereck J, Kumarswamy R, Foinquinos A, Xiao K, Avramopoulos P, Kunz M, et al. Long noncoding RNA Chast promotes cardiac remodeling. Sci Transl Med 2016;8:326ra22. DOI:10.1126/scitranslmed.aaf1475.

[85] Huang S, Li X, Zheng H, Si X, Li B, Wei G, et al. Loss of Super-Enhancer-Regulated circRNA Nfix Induces Cardiac Regeneration After Myocardial Infarction in Adult Mice. Circulation 2019;139:2857-2876. DOI:10.1161/CIRCULATIONAHA.118.038361.

[86] Park I-H, Erbay E, Nuzzi P, Chen J. Skeletal myocyte hypertrophy requires mTOR kinase activity and S6K1. Exp Cell Res 2005;309:211-219. DOI:10.1016/j.yexcr.2005.05.017.

[87] Schulze PC, Gielen S, Schuler G, Hambrecht R. Chronic heart failure and skeletal muscle catabolism: effects of exercise training. Int J Cardiol 2002;85:141-149. DOI:10.1016/s0167-5273(02)00243-7.

[88] Egan B, Zierath JR. Exercise metabolism and the molecular regulation of skeletal muscle adaptation. Cell Metab 2013;17:162-184. DOI:10.1016/j.cmet.2012.12.012.

[89] Bueno CR, Ferreira JCB, Pereira MG, Bacurau AVN, Brum PC. Aerobic exercise training improves skeletal muscle function and Ca2+ handling-related protein expression in sympathetic hyperactivity-induced heart failure. J Appl Physiol 2010;109:702-709. DOI:10.1152/japplphysiol.00281.2010.

[90] Bodine SC. mTOR signaling and the molecular adaptation to resistance

exercise. Med Sci Sports Exerc 2006;38:1950-1957. DOI:10.1249/01. mss.0000233797.24035.35.

[91] Zhao J, Brault JJ, Schild A, Cao P, Sandri M, Schiaffino S, et al. FoxO3 coordinately activates protein degradation by the autophagic/ lysosomal and proteasomal pathways in atrophying muscle cells. Cell Metab 2007;6:472-483. DOI:10.1016/j. cmet.2007.11.004.

[92] Ren J, Samson WK, Sowers JR. Insulin-like growth factor I as a cardiac hormone: physiological and pathophysiological implications in heart disease. J Mol Cell Cardiol 1999;31:2049-2061. DOI:10.1006/ jmcc.1999.1036.

[93] Da Costa Martins PA, De Windt LJ. MicroRNAs in control of cardiac hypertrophy. Cardiovasc Res 2012;93:563-572. DOI:10.1093/ cvr/cvs013.

[94] Lim TB, Aliwarga E, Luu TDA, Li YP, Ng SL, Annadoray L, et al. Targeting the highly abundant circular RNA circSlc8a1 in cardiomyocytes attenuates pressure overload induced hypertrophy. Cardiovasc Res 2019;115:1998-2007. DOI:10.1093/ cvr/cvz130.

[95] Elia L, Contu R, Quintavalle M, Varrone F, Chimenti C, Russo MA, et al. Reciprocal regulation of microRNA-1 and insulin-like growth factor-1 signal transduction cascade in cardiac and skeletal muscle in physiological and pathological conditions. Circulation 2009;120:2377-2385. DOI:10.1161/ CIRCULATIONAHA.109.879429.

[96] Huang M-B, Xu H, Xie S-J, Zhou H, Qu L-H. Insulin-like growth factor-1 receptor is regulated by microRNA-133 during skeletal myogenesis. PLoS One 2011;6:e29173. DOI:10.1371/journal. pone.0029173.

[97] Ganesan J, Ramanujam D, Sassi Y, Ahles A, Jentzsch C, Werfel S, et al. MiR-378 controls cardiac hypertrophy by combined repression of mitogen- activated protein kinase pathway factors. Circulation 2013;127:2097-2106. DOI:10.1161/CIRCULATIONAHA. 112.000882.

[98] Antunes-Correa LM, Trevizan PF, Bacurau AVN, Ferreira-Santos L, Gomes JLP, Urias U, et al. Effects of aerobic and inspiratory training on skeletal muscle microRNA-1 and downstream-associated pathways in patients with heart failure. J Cachexia Sarcopenia Muscle 2020;11:89-102. DOI:10.1002/jcsm.12495.

[99] Xu X-D, Song X-W, Li Q, Wang G-K, Jing Q, Qin Y-W. Attenuation of microRNA-22 derepressed PTEN to effectively protect rat cardiomyocytes from hypertrophy. J Cell Physiol 2012;227:1391-1398. DOI:10.1002/ jcp.22852.

[100] Huang Z-P, Chen J, Seok HY, Zhang Z, Kataoka M, Hu X, et al. MicroRNA-22 regulates cardiac hypertrophy and remodeling in response to stress. Circ Res 2013;112:1234-1243. DOI:10.1161/ CIRCRESAHA.112.300682.

[101] Sassi Y, Avramopoulos P, Ramanujam D, Grüter L, Werfel S, Giosele S, et al. Cardiac myocyte miR-29 promotes pathological remodeling of the heart by activating Wnt signaling. Nat Commun 2017;8:1614. DOI:10.1038/ s41467-017-01737-4.

[102] Wang K, Lin Z-Q, Long B, Li J-H, Zhou J, Li P-F. Cardiac hypertrophy is positively regulated by MicroRNA miR-23a. J Biol Chem 2012;287:589-599. DOI:10.1074/jbc.M111.266940.

[103] Ucar A, Gupta SK, Fiedler J, Erikci E, Kardasinski M, Batkai S, et al. The miRNA-212/132 family regulates both cardiac hypertrophy and

cardiomyocyte autophagy. Nat Commun 2012;3:1078. DOI:10.1038/ncomms2090.

[104] Wang K, Long B, Liu F, Wang J-X, Liu C-Y, Zhao B, et al. A circular RNA protects the heart from pathological hypertrophy and heart failure by targeting miR-223. Eur Heart J 2016;37:2602-2611. DOI:10.1093/eurheartj/ehv713.

[105] Fabbri M, Paone A, Calore F, Galli R, Gaudio E, Santhanam R, et al. MicroRNAs bind to Toll-like receptors to induce prometastatic inflammatory response. Proc Natl Acad Sci 2012;109:E2110–E2116. DOI:10.1073/pnas.1209414109.

[106] He WA, Calore F, Londhe P, Canella A, Guttridge DC, Croce CM. Microvesicles containing miRNAs promote muscle cell death in cancer cachexia via TLR7. Proc Natl Acad Sci 2014;111:4525-4529. DOI:10.1073/pnas.1402714111.

[107] Freire PP, Fernandez GJ, Cury SS, de Moraes D, Oliveira JS, de Oliveira G, et al. The Pathway to Cancer Cachexia: MicroRNA-Regulated Networks in Muscle Wasting Based on Integrative Meta-Analysis. Int J Mol Sci 2019;20:1962. DOI:10.3390/ijms20081962.

[108] Chacon-Cabrera A, Fermoselle C, Salmela I, Yelamos J, Barreiro E. MicroRNA expression and protein acetylation pattern in respiratory and limb muscles of Parp-1−/− and Parp-2−/− mice with lung cancer cachexia. Biochim Biophys Acta - Gen Subj 2015;1850:2530-2543. DOI:10.1016/j.bbagen.2015.09.020.

[109] Lee DE, Brown JL, Rosa-Caldwell ME, Blackwell TA, Perry RA, Brown LA, et al. Cancer cachexia-induced muscle atrophy: evidence for alterations in microRNAs important for muscle size. Physiol Genomics 2017;49:253-260.

DOI:10.1152/physiolgenomics.00006.2017.

[110] Kulyté A, Lorente-Cebrián S, Gao H, Mejhert N, Agustsson T, Arner P, et al. MicroRNA profiling links miR-378 to enhanced adipocyte lipolysis in human cancer cachexia. Am J Physiol Endocrinol Metab 2014;306:E267-E274. DOI:10.1152/ajpendo.00249.2013.

[111] Narasimhan A, Ghosh S, Stretch C, Greiner R, Bathe OF, Baracos V, et al. Small RNAome profiling from human skeletal muscle: novel miRNAs and their targets associated with cancer cachexia. J Cachexia Sarcopenia Muscle 2017;8:405-416. DOI:10.1002/jcsm.12168.

[112] Worp WRPH, Schols AMWJ, Dingemans AC, Op den Kamp CMH, Degens JHRJ, Kelders MCJM, et al. Identification of microRNAs in skeletal muscle associated with lung cancer cachexia. J Cachexia Sarcopenia Muscle 2020;11:452-463. DOI:10.1002/jcsm.12512.

[113] Li Z, Cai B, Abdalla BA, Zhu X, Zheng M, Han P, et al. LncIRS1 controls muscle atrophy via sponging miR-15 family to activate IGF1-PI3K/AKT pathway. J Cachexia Sarcopenia Muscle 2019;10:391-410. DOI:10.1002/jcsm.12374.

[114] Zhang Z-K, Li J, Guan D, Liang C, Zhuo Z, Liu J, et al. A newly identified lncRNA MAR1 acts as a miR-487b sponge to promote skeletal muscle differentiation and regeneration. J Cachexia Sarcopenia Muscle 2018;9:613-626. DOI:10.1002/jcsm.12281.

[115] Shen L, Han J, Wang H, Meng Q, Chen L, Liu Y, et al. Cachexia-related long noncoding RNA, CAAlnc1, suppresses adipogenesis by blocking the binding of HuR to adipogenic transcription factor mRNAs. Int J Cancer 2019;145:1809-1821. DOI:10.1002/ijc.32236.

[116] Gong C, Li Z, Ramanujan K, Clay I, Zhang Y, Lemire-Brachat S, et al. A long non-coding RNA, LncMyoD, regulates skeletal muscle differentiation by blocking IMP2-mediated mRNA translation. Dev Cell 2015;34:181-191. DOI:10.1016/j.devcel.2015.05.009.

[117] Han J, Shen L, Zhan Z, Liu Y, Zhang C, Guo R, et al. The long noncoding RNA MALAT1 modulates adipose loss in cancer-associated cachexia by suppressing adipogenesis through PPAR-γ. Nutr Metab (Lond) 2021;18:27. DOI:10.1186/s12986-021-00557-0.

[118] Zhang H, Zhu L, Bai M, Liu Y, Zhan Y, Deng T, et al. Exosomal circRNA derived from gastric tumor promotes white adipose browning by targeting the miR-133/PRDM16 pathway. Int J Cancer 2019;144:2501-2515. DOI:10.1002/ijc.31977.

[119] Roh J, Rhee J, Chaudhari V, Rosenzweig A. The Role of Exercise in Cardiac Aging: From Physiology to Molecular Mechanisms. Circ Res 2016;118:279-295. DOI:10.1161/CIRCRESAHA.115.305250.

[120] Wang H, Liang Y, Li Y. Non-coding RNAs in exercise. Non-Coding RNA Investig 2017;1:10-10. DOI:10.21037/ncri.2017.09.01.

[121] Liu Y, Hu F, Li D, Wang F, Zhu L, Chen W, et al. Does physical activity reduce the risk of prostate cancer? A systematic review and meta-analysis. Eur Urol 2011;60:1029-1044. DOI:10.1016/j.eururo.2011.07.007.

[122] Passantino A, Dalla Vecchia LA, Corrà U, Scalvini S, Pistono M, Bussotti M, et al. The Future of Exercise-Based Cardiac Rehabilitation for Patients With Heart Failure. Front Cardiovasc Med 2021;8:709898. DOI:10.3389/fcvm.2021.709898.

[123] Brown BM, Peiffer JJ, Martins RN. Multiple effects of physical activity on molecular and cognitive signs of brain aging: can exercise slow neurodegeneration and delay Alzheimer's disease? Mol Psychiatry 2013;18:864-874. DOI:10.1038/mp.2012.162.

[124] Bozkurt B, Hershberger RE, Butler J, Grady KL, Heidenreich PA, Isler ML, et al. 2021 ACC/AHA Key Data Elements and Definitions for Heart Failure: A Report of the American College of Cardiology/American Heart Association Task Force on Clinical Data Standards (Writing Committee to Develop Clinical Data Standards for Heart Failure). Circ Cardiovasc Qual Outcomes 2021;14:e000102. DOI:10.1161/HCQ.0000000000000102.

[125] Rock CL, Thomson C, Gansler T, Gapstur SM, McCullough ML, Patel A V, et al. American Cancer Society guideline for diet and physical activity for cancer prevention. CA Cancer J Clin 2020;70:245-271. DOI:10.3322/caac.21591.

[126] Brum PC, Bacurau A V, Cunha TF, Bechara LRG, Moreira JBN. Skeletal myopathy in heart failure: effects of aerobic exercise training. Exp Physiol 2014;99:616-620. DOI:10.1113/expphysiol.2013.076844.

[127] Drummond MJ. MicroRNAs and exercise-induced skeletal muscle adaptations. J Physiol 2010;588:3849-3850. DOI:10.1113/jphysiol.2010.198218.

[128] Ellison GM, Waring CD, Vicinanza C, Torella D. Physiological cardiac remodelling in response to endurance exercise training: cellular and molecular mechanisms. Heart 2012;98:5-10. DOI:10.1136/heartjnl-2011-300639.

[129] Lin H, Zhu Y, Zheng C, Hu D, Ma S, Chen L, et al. Antihypertrophic Memory After Regression of Exercise-Induced Physiological Myocardial Hypertrophy Is Mediated by the Long

Noncoding RNA Mhrt779. Circulation 2021;143:2277-2292. DOI:10.1161/CIRCULATIONAHA.120.047000.

[130] Aoi W. Frontier impact of microRNAs in skeletal muscle research: a future perspective. Front Physiol 2014;5:495. DOI:10.3389/fphys.2014.00495.

[131] Bonilauri B, Dallagiovanna B. Long Non-coding RNAs Are Differentially Expressed After Different Exercise Training Programs. Front Physiol 2020;11:567614. DOI:10.3389/fphys.2020.567614.

[132] Guo M, Qiu J, Shen F, Wang S, Yu J, Zuo H, et al. Comprehensive analysis of circular RNA profiles in skeletal muscles of aging mice and after aerobic exercise intervention. Aging (Albany NY) 2020;12:5071-90. DOI:10.18632/aging.102932.

[133] Meinecke A, Mitzka S, Just A, Cushman S, Stojanović SD, Xiao K, et al. Cardiac endurance training alters plasma profiles of circular RNA MBOAT2. Am J Physiol Heart Circ Physiol 2020;319:H13–H21. DOI:10.1152/ajpheart.00067.2020.

[134] Negrao CE, Middlekauff HR, Gomes-Santos IL, Antunes-Correa LM. Effects of exercise training on neurovascular control and skeletal myopathy in systolic heart failure. Am J Physiol Heart Circ Physiol 2015;308:H792-H802. DOI:10.1152/ajpheart.00830.2014.

[135] Campos JC, Queliconi BB, Bozi LHM, Bechara LRG, Dourado PMM, Andres AM, et al. Exercise reestablishes autophagic flux and mitochondrial quality control in heart failure. Autophagy 2017;13:1304-1317. DOI:10.1080/15548627.2017.1325062.

[136] Adamopoulos S, Coats AJ, Brunotte F, Arnolda L, Meyer T, Thompson CH, et al. Physical training improves skeletal muscle metabolism in patients with chronic heart failure. J Am Coll Cardiol 1993;21:1101-1106. DOI:10.1016/0735-1097(93)90231-o.

[137] Linke A, Adams V, Schulze PC, Erbs S, Gielen S, Fiehn E, et al. Antioxidative effects of exercise training in patients with chronic heart failure: increase in radical scavenger enzyme activity in skeletal muscle. Circulation 2005;111:1763-1770. DOI:10.1161/01.CIR.0000165503.08661.E5.

[138] Gielen S, Adams V, Möbius-Winkler S, Linke A, Erbs S, Yu J, et al. Anti-inflammatory effects of exercise training in the skeletal muscle of patients with chronic heart failure. J Am Coll Cardiol 2003;42:861-868. DOI:10.1016/s0735-1097(03)00848-9.

[139] Wang L, Lv Y, Li G, Xiao J. MicroRNAs in heart and circulation during physical exercise. J Sport Heal Sci 2018;7:433-441. DOI:10.1016/j.jshs.2018.09.008.

[140] Fernandes T, Baraúna VG, Negrão CE, Phillips MI, Oliveira EM. Aerobic exercise training promotes physiological cardiac remodeling involving a set of microRNAs. Am J Physiol Heart Circ Physiol 2015;309:H543-H552. DOI:10.1152/ajpheart.00899.2014.

[141] Souza RWA, Fernandez GJ, Cunha JPQ, Piedade WP, Soares LC, Souza PAT, et al. Regulation of cardiac microRNAs induced by aerobic exercise training during heart failure. Am J Physiol Heart Circ Physiol 2015;309:H1629-H1641. DOI:10.1152/ajpheart.00941.2014.

[142] Carè A, Catalucci D, Felicetti F, Bonci D, Addario A, Gallo P, et al. MicroRNA-133 controls cardiac hypertrophy. Nat Med 2007;13:613-618. DOI:10.1038/nm1582.

[143] Shi J, Bei Y, Kong X, Liu X, Lei Z, Xu T, et al. miR-17-3p Contributes to Exercise-Induced Cardiac Growth and Protects against Myocardial Ischemia-Reperfusion Injury. Theranostics 2017;7:664-676. DOI:10.7150/thno. 15162.

[144] Baggish AL, Park J, Min P-K, Isaacs S, Parker BA, Thompson PD, et al. Rapid upregulation and clearance of distinct circulating microRNAs after prolonged aerobic exercise. J Appl Physiol 2014;116:522-531. DOI:10.1152/japplphysiol.01141.2013.

[145] Aoi W, Ichikawa H, Mune K, Tanimura Y, Mizushima K, Naito Y, et al. Muscle-enriched microRNA miR-486 decreases in circulation in response to exercise in young men. Front Physiol 2013;4:80. DOI:10.3389/fphys.2013. 00080.

[146] Leal LG, Lopes MA, Peres SB, Batista ML. Exercise Training as Therapeutic Approach in Cancer Cachexia: A Review of Potential Anti-inflammatory Effect on Muscle Wasting. Front Physiol 2021;11. DOI:10.3389/fphys.2020.570170.

[147] Maddocks M, Murton AJ, Wilcock A. Therapeutic exercise in cancer cachexia. Crit Rev Oncog 2012;17:285-292. DOI:10.1615/critrevoncog.v17.i3.60.

[148] Grande AJ, Silva V, Sawaris Neto L, Teixeira Basmage JP, Peccin MS, Maddocks M. Exercise for cancer cachexia in adults. Cochrane Database Syst Rev 2021;2021. DOI:10.1002/14651858.CD010804.pub3.

[149] Donatto FF, Neves RX, Rosa FO, Camargo RG, Ribeiro H, Matos-Neto EM, et al. Resistance exercise modulates lipid plasma profile and cytokine content in the adipose tissue of tumour-bearing rats. Cytokine 2013;61:426-432. DOI:10.1016/j. cyto.2012.10.021.

[150] Pedersen BK, Fischer CP. Beneficial health effects of exercise--the role of IL-6 as a myokine. Trends Pharmacol Sci 2007;28:152-156. DOI:10.1016/j. tips.2007.02.002.

[151] Pedersen L, Idorn M, Olofsson GH, Lauenborg B, Nookaew I, Hansen RH, et al. Voluntary Running Suppresses Tumor Growth through Epinephrine- and IL-6-Dependent NK Cell Mobilization and Redistribution. Cell Metab 2016;23:554-562. DOI:10.1016/j. cmet.2016.01.011.

[152] Pigna E, Berardi E, Aulino P, Rizzuto E, Zampieri S, Carraro U, et al. Aerobic Exercise and Pharmacological Treatments Counteract Cachexia by Modulating Autophagy in Colon Cancer. Sci Rep 2016;6:26991. DOI:10.1038/srep26991.

[153] Ballarò R, Beltrà M, De Lucia S, Pin F, Ranjbar K, Hulmi JJ, et al. Moderate exercise in mice improves cancer plus chemotherapy-induced muscle wasting and mitochondrial alterations. FASEB J 2019;33:5482-5494. DOI:10.1096/fj.201801862R.

[154] Padilha CS, Cella PS, Chimin P, Voltarelli FA, Marinello PC, de Jesus Testa MT, et al. Resistance Training's Ability to Prevent Cancer-induced Muscle Atrophy Extends Anabolic Stimulus. Med Sci Sport Exerc 2021;Publish Ah. DOI:10.1249/MSS.0000000000002624.

[155] Tanaka M, Sugimoto K, Fujimoto T, Xie K, Takahashi T, Akasaka H, et al. Preventive effects of low-intensity exercise on cancer cachexia–induced muscle atrophy. FASEB J 2019;33:7852-7862. DOI:10.1096/fj.201802430R.

[156] Powrózek T, Mlak R, Brzozowska A, Mazurek M, Gołębiowski P, Małecka-Massalska T. miRNA-130a Significantly Improves Accuracy of SGA Nutritional Assessment Tool in Prediction of

Malnutrition and Cachexia in Radiotherapy-Treated Head and Neck Cancer Patients. Cancers (Basel) 2018;10. DOI:10.3390/cancers10090294.

[157] Okugawa Y, Yao L, Toiyama Y, Yamamoto A, Shigemori T, Yin C, et al. Prognostic impact of sarcopenia and its correlation with circulating miR-21 in colorectal cancer patients. Oncol Rep 2018;39:1555-1564. DOI:10.3892/or.2018.6270.

[158] Okugawa Y, Toiyama Y, Hur K, Yamamoto A, Yin C, Ide S, et al. Circulating miR-203 derived from metastatic tissues promotes myopenia in colorectal cancer patients. J Cachexia Sarcopenia Muscle 2019;10:536-548. DOI:10.1002/jcsm.12403.

[159] Chen D, Goswami CP, Burnett RM, Anjanappa M, Bhat-Nakshatri P, Muller W, et al. Cancer Affects microRNA Expression, Release, and Function in Cardiac and Skeletal Muscle. Cancer Res 2014;74:4270-4281. DOI:10.1158/0008-5472.CAN-13-2817.

[160] Zhang C, Yao C, Li H, Wang G, He X. Serum levels of microRNA-133b and microRNA-206 expression predict prognosis in patients with osteosarcoma. Int J Clin Exp Pathol 2014;7:4194-4203.

[161] Nohata N, Hanazawa T, Enokida H, Seki N. microRNA-1/133a and microRNA-206/133b clusters: dysregulation and functional roles in human cancers. Oncotarget 2012;3:9-21. DOI:10.18632/oncotarget.424.

[162] Hu Z, Chen X, Zhao Y, Tian T, Jin G, Shu Y, et al. Serum microRNA signatures identified in a genome-wide serum microRNA expression profiling predict survival of non-small-cell lung cancer. J Clin Oncol 2010;28:1721-1726. DOI:10.1200/JCO.2009.24.9342.

Chapter 7

Combined Ketogenic Diet and Walking Exercise Interventions in Community Older Frailty and Skeletal Muscle Sarcopenia

Jia-Ping Wu

Abstract

The ketogenic diet and walking exercise training interventions are two key public health lifestyle factors. The potential of combined lifestyle factors interventions focused on getting to compliance in diet and exercise. A balanced ketogenic diet and regular exercise interventions is key modifiable factor to the prevention and management of community older frailty and skeletal muscle sarcopenia. Influence health across the lifespan and reduction of the risk of premature death through several biochemistry mechanisms. Community older group's lifestyle factors interventions contribute identity in their natural living environment. While the older health benefits of walking exercise training interventions strategies are commonly to study, combining ketogenic diet and walking exercise interventions can induce greater benefits in community older groups.

Keywords: ketogenic diet, exercise therapy, community health planning, natural, exercise intervention

1. Introduction

The ketogenic diet is a 60% high-fat, 30% adequate-protein, and 10% low-carbohydrate diet used to treat aging-related diseases in the community older groups. The ketogenic diet interventions are a specialized diet that involves a highly restricted intake of carbohydrates and proteins and a high proportion of fat consumption in community older groups [1]. It has proven to be used in the treatment of older-related diseases in community groups because the mechanism of action of the ketogenic diet interventions causes changes in the levels of ketone bodies with exercise training interventions in the body, reducing the aging-related diseases [2, 3]. The purpose of this chapter review was to systematically review the systemic effects of ketogenic diet restriction when combined with walking exercise intervention in community older groups. Thus, in this chapter review, we want to discuss combining ketogenic diet interventions and walking exercise interventions in community older groups. The ketogenic diets very high in fat can promote ketogenesis differently depending on other different macronutrient ratios [4]. The ketogenic diets intervention for weight loss in older humans may be counterproductive to obesity, however, which is not typically associated with

NAFLD/NASH [5, 6]. Acetoacetate, acetone, and β-hydroxybutyrate are the three ketone bodies produced in community older groups. It is also important to eat healthy ketogenic diet interventions and exercise interventions regularly as well as a check-in with your healthcare provider [7]. After a short-time walking exercise, make appropriate adjustments based on your own feelings, such as frailty and sleepiness [8]. However, the benefits of walking exercise regimens improve the immune system, helps digestion, promote the release of muscle hormones, and when they enter the body to eliminate inflammation, reduce visceral fat, reduce inflammation, helps improve brain-derived neurotrophic factor substances, mitochondrial cells work normally, and help longevity [9]. The precise regimen of action of the combined ketogenic diet interventions and walking exercise interventions in community older groups is not known, although many possible interventions explanations have been proposed. There are many changes that occur in the body as a result of the ketogenic diet, but it is unclear which of these alterations is responsible for the walking exercise interventions effects. This is expected, however, as the mechanism of action of the combined ketogenic diet and walking exercise interventions in community older groups is similarly a mystery [10]. Sarcopenia and frailty are prevalent in the community of older aging-related diseases [11]. Sarcopenia is because of the presence of loss of muscle mass with low muscle strength and low physical function in the community older groups (**Figure 1**). What is sarcopenia? And what causes sarcopenia?

Sarcopenia is defined as the loss of both coordination of muscle mass and strength, which causes difficulty walking and poor daily activities balance. Sarcopenia is a major aging-related disease with a health condition for contributes to public health and sociate. Aging-related skeletal muscle sarcopenia can lead to disability and lack of independence, as well as increase the risk of falls. Skeletal muscle strength loss led to lower muscle function (**Figure 1A**), and skeletal muscle structure disruption, in addition to a loss of muscle mass because of an increase in fat tissue skeletal muscle strength evaluated appendicular muscle mass was measured with dual-energy X-ray absorptiometry (**Figure 1B**). Aging disrupts skeletal muscle ability to lose maintain muscles. With aging, a lot of signals are sent from the brain to the muscle leading to a loss in mass and strong (**Figure 2A**). Frailty is a body system impairment associated with increased oxygen stressor. The walking exercise interventions regimens are to stave off frailty transitions over time among

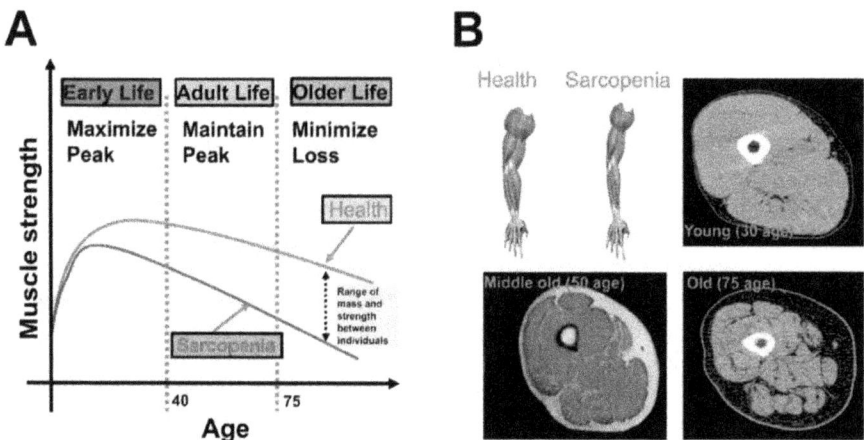

Figure 1.
Sarcopenia is a muscle-wasting condition disease. (A) Skeletal muscle strength loss is related to aging. (B). Skeletal muscle structure disruption is associated with aging.

A   **B**

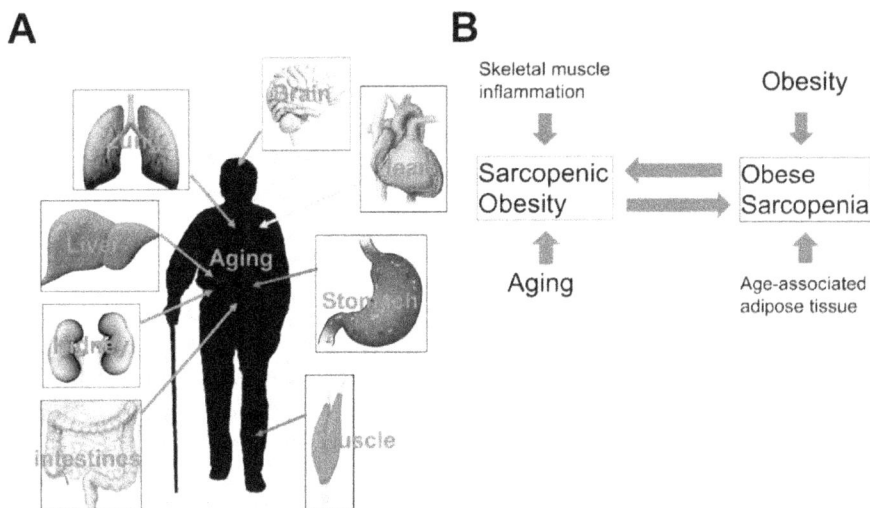

Figure 2.
Combined ketogenic diet and exercise interventions in community older groups. (A) The foods of the ketogenic diet we eat can support or hinder older health. The different intensity exercise interventions combined with the ketogenic diet have different effects on the older man's health. (B) Obese sarcopenia can contribute to obesity-induced muscle loss. Aging-related sarcopenia contributes to age-induced muscle loss.

the elderly populations [12]. Both sarcopenia and frailty are detrimental outcomes in older adults to processes exacerbated by acute illness or injury. Multiple weight cycles in the community older groups are a predictor of lower muscle mass and reduced strength with potential for sarcopenia in elderly with obesity (**Figure 2B**). Severe obesity overweight cyclers with lower muscle mass and strength showed a greater risk of developing sarcopenia. Pro-inflammation is a hallmark of aging. Aging-associated obesity is adipose tissue and skeletal muscle inflammation associated with skeletal muscle loss and impaired myogenesis [13]. Combined ketogenic diet interventions and walking exercise interventions are shown to decline infiltration of proinflammatory macrophages in skeletal muscle sarcopenia in obesity and being associated with muscle insulin resistance in the community human older groups.

2. The ketogenic diet in the community older skeletal muscle sarcopenia

The key aspect of the ketogenic diet is a high proportion of fats, adequate levels of protein, a low proportion of carbohydrates primarily used to treatment difficult-to-control aging chronic diseases [14]. The ketogenic diet is now used to treat in the community older groups for rapidly burning more fat when there is a low carbohydrate intake [15]. The ketogenic diet, low carbohydrate intake, can lead to elevated blood ketone bodies. Measured blood ketones levels can allow for adjustment of the ketogenic diet to meet the user's needs [16]. But now new technologies are being researched in the breath acetone sensors are becoming more popular due to less invasiveness and convenience [17–19]. Future technologies are very promising but are still in the early development stages. The ketogenic diet became popular as a therapy for epilepsy in the 1920s and 30s. Recently, it was developed to provide an alternative to anti-aging, which had demonstrated success as an aging therapy [20]. However, the ketogenic diet interventions are eventually largely abandoned due to the mitochondrial dysfunction and excessive inflammatory responses to induce pathology in age-related diseases in the community older groups. There are several theories about the mechanism of action of the ketogenic diet intervention including increased acidity in the blood.

2.1 The Ketogenic diet is converted to ketone bodies

The ketogenic diets forces to burn off of fats rather than carbohydrates [21]. A ketogenic diet, a high fat, in food is converted triglyceride (TG). The liver converts triacylglycerol (TAG) into fatty acid and ketone bodies. An elevated ketone body in the blood eventually lowers the aging-related diseases [22]. We hoped that keto-genic diet therapy could be maintained ketone bodies by the liver in the community older groups. Blood ketone bodies were produced β-hydroxybutyrate, acetoacetate, and acetone. They consumed a very low-carbohydrate, and excess high-fat diet [23]. Ketone bodies (KBs) are considered as an alternative source of energy supply [24]. When a person eats a regular ketogenic diet, food is converted into glucose, which is transported around the body and used by various cells as an energy source [25], but when too little carbohydrates are available, the liver processes fats to provide the brain with energy in the form of fatty acids and ketone bodies. An increased blood level of ketone bodies is referred to as ketosis. These ketone bodies are thought to possess anti-aging properties in the community older groups, as β-hydroxybutyrate supplementary has been shown to protect old human health [26]. In 1921, endo-crinologists demonstrated that ketone bodies were produced by the liver including three water-soluble compounds, acetone, β-hydroxybutyrate, and acetoacetate, as they eat a diet rich in fat and low in carbohydrates.

The key aspect of the ketogenic diet involves the restriction of carbohydrates, which are no longer able to be converted to glucose and provide for the body's metabolic and energy needs . To compensate for this, fatty acids are converted into fuel sources through a process of oxidation in the mitochondria. To detect acetoac-etate in blood, but does not react with β-hydroxybutyrate which is the predominant circulating ketone body. In the community older groups' bodies can become more strongly positive as the metabolic derangements improve β-hydroxybutyrate is con-verted to acetoacetate . The ketogenic diet mimics aspects of starvation, the body is forced to burn fats rather than carbohydrates, when this is combined with a low intake of carbohydrates which causes the body to produce ketones . The stabiliza-tion of the ketogenic diet may occur as a result of the efficiency of the ketone bodies as a fuel source. The ketogenic diet is converted fatty acids to ketone bodies for energy to increase the number of mitochondria as the body adapts [27]. However, this is of no consequence provided the ketogenic diet converted ketone bodies (β-hydroxybutyrate and acetoacetate) are closing in community older groups and the patient is continuing to improve clinically (**Figure 3A**).

2.2 The β-hydroxybutyrate (BHB) ketone supplements interventions in the community older skeletal muscle sarcopenia

It is not surprising that sarcopenia obesity or obese sarcopenia is linked to many adverse health outcomes, such as ketogenic diet and exercise training. Thus, skeletal muscle is the largest organ making up around 40% of body weight. It is essential for metabolic functions regulating blood glucose levels in the body. Furthermore, we discuss the role of β-hydroxybutyrate (BHB) supplementary interventions exercise factors released by the liver [28]. Walking exercise training may be able to increase their blood β-hydroxybutyrate (BHB) concentrations in the community older groups and be increased in ketosis. Endogenous production of high levels of the ketone body β-hydroxybutyrate (BHB) is regarded as 5 mM blood BHB for

A   **B**

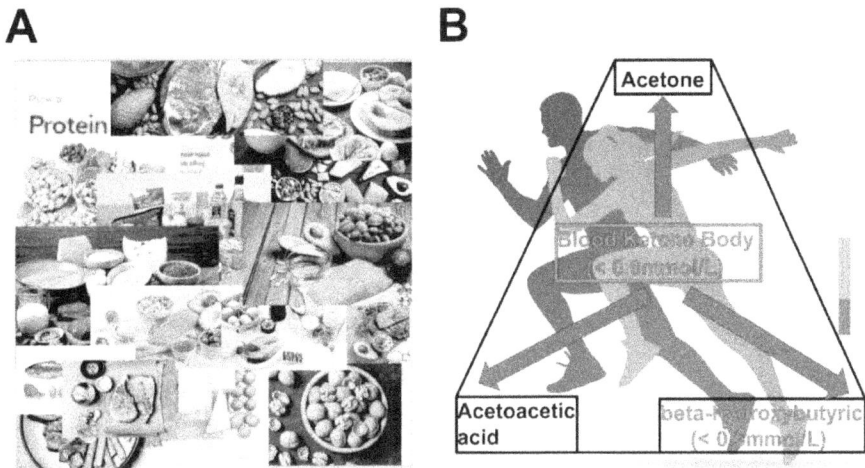

Figure 3.
The ketone body converses. (A) The ketogenic diet foods. (B) Ketogenic diet raised ketone body levels. Blood ketone bodies (<0.6 mmole/L) are markers specifically β-hydroxybutyrate (BHB), acetoacetate (AcAc), and acetone. The breath acetone level is lower compared to blood BHB. Direct measurement of beta-hydroxybutyrate circumvents this problem. Therefore, the β-hydroxybutyrate (BHB) blood test may underestimate the true circulating ketone bodies.

120 min after walking exercise in the older men (**Figure 3B**) [29]. This ketogenic diet has long been used as a treatment in the community of older men focused on the therapeutic effects of the ketone body β-hydroxybutyrate (BHB). Recent reports demonstrate that developed ketone can help significantly increase the blood circulating β-hydroxybutyrate in the community older humans [30]. Ketone supplements can efficiently attenuate age-related diseases in older humans. We argue this inflection point affects older human health. Some reports indicated that one of the ketone bodies, β-hydroxybutyrate (BHB), in the community older humans can inhibit aging-related diseases, such as sarcopenia or Alzheimer's disease (AD) . The favorable aspect of ketosis in both ketogenic diet and ketogenic supplements in aging-related diseases has been discussed. We summarize and suggest that aging research is entering a new milestone that has unique medical, commercial, and societal implications.

2.3 The different types of ketogenic diet intervention regimens in the community older skeletal muscle sarcopenia

Many foods and drugs used to treat these conditions can contribute to sarcopenia, as they can cause an imbalance in muscle metabolic and disrupt the pathways that control muscle mass. Nutritional ketogenic diet factors are also important for maintaining muscle and muscle growth in community older patients who may be sarcopenia and frailty. With an adequate intake of protein each day, most people should aim to lean meat, poultry, fish, seafood, eggs, nuts, seeds, and legumes (**Figure 2A**). The ketogenic diet intervention regimens are a special diet designed to help the community older groups that fail to respond adequately to aging-related diseases [31]. In the absence of glucose due to lack of carbohydrates in the ketogenic diet interventions, the community older groups are no longer able to be converted to glucose and provide the body's metabolic and energy needs, fatty acids are the majored converted into the fuel sources through synthesized the ketone bodies β-hydroxybutyrate, acetoacetate and acetone [32, 33]. The ketogenic diet is a mixed diet containing low carbohydrates, consisting primarily of proteins and fat. Some healthy foods are eaten on a ketogenic diet, for example, seafood, low-carb vegetables, cheese, eggs, meat, poultry, coffee, and tea (**Figure 3A**) [34]. The importance of high fat in aging-related diseases reducing regimens on different walking exercise training models is shown by comparing the effects of four different types of ketogenic dietary regimens. A typical ketogenic diet interventions regimens are made up of the following: (I). A standard keto diet (SKD): typically contains a very low, only 5% carbohydrate, 15% moderate proteins, and 80% high fat diet. This classic SKD contains a 3:1 ratio to combined protein and carbohydrate. (II) The high protein keto diet (HPKD): this contains 5% carbohydrates, 35% protein, and 60% fat. HPKD is about the same as the standard keto diet but includes more protein. (III) The cyclical keto diet (CKD): this ketogenic diet feeds like 5 ketogenic days of periods of higher-carbs feeds, and then 2 high carbohydrate days. (IV) The targeted keto diet (TKD): this type of ketogenic diet allows you to add more around carbohydrates workouts. Although this keto diet is usually safe for diabetes, epilepsy, and aging-related diseases, they may be had some initial body adaptation. Be sure to consume a balanced optimized ketogenic diet to support your fitness program. All food groups are necessary to sustain healthy energy levels and get the most out of your workout [35]. A ketogenic diet contains 5% carbohydrates, carbohydrates are vital, as they can fuel your muscles before exercise [36]. Carbohydrates are also important after walking exercise training to replenish glycogen stores and assist with the absorption of amino acids into your muscles during recovery [37]. Up to 35% protein helps to improve muscle recovery after walking exercise training, repairs tissue damage, and builds muscle mass [38]. Up to 60% of consuming healthy fats has been shown to help burn body fat and preserve muscle fuel during workouts, making your energy last longer [39]. The ketogenic diet interventions contain adequate amounts of protein for body growth. The total protein in the ketogenic diet is also sufficient to maintain health for a given older age. In the classic ketogenic diet, the ratio of fats to carbohydrates and proteins combined is 4:1 [40]. Although it emerged in the community older groups of aging-related diseases could be effectively controlled using these interventions. They may still fail to achieve aging control in the community older groups [41]. For these intervention individuals, the ketogenic diet interventions were re-introduced as a technique for managing the condition. However, the ketogenic diet has been shown in a study of rats to have anti-aging properties and inhibit the development of aging-related diseases in the community older groups.

3. The walking exercise intervention in the community older skeletal muscle sarcopenia

What causes of sarcopenia in community older people? By the age of 70, sarcopenia affects 10–30% of older adults lost muscle mass and this is replaced with fat and fibrous tissue, particularly in people who are physical inactivity, malnutrition, hormones changes, inflammation increased, and aging-related diseases. Sarcopenia is common in older people, but can also earlier in their 40s life without exercise intervention causes skeletal muscle mass and strength begin to decline and accelerate with aging [42]. Exercise training can help lower the risk of aging-related diseases in the older community groups, for example, decreases blood pressure, lower LDL cholesterol levels, developing type 2 diabetes, increase your heart's size and strength, and improve cardiorespiratory fitness. Walking exercise training is a low-intensity aerobic activity that reduces the risk of the older community groups' diseases [43]. If you have another aging-related chronic disease, you should speak with your healthcare professional before starting a new exercise program. The difference of intensity of walking exercise performs change arterial system during the exercise stimulus [44]. Moderate walking exercise training models can improve arterial endothelial function in the community group of an older healthy man. General recommendations to promote good overall health, aim to get at least 150 min of moderate-intensity exercise, or 75 min of high-intensity exercise training, or a combination of the two each week for optimal young adult health [45]. However, low-intensity walking exercise training for 15 min at least three times per week and spend 10 min of your lunch break walking exercise. Chronic exercise training that can mimic the effects of exercise is associated with lower blood pressure response in older men [46]. Starting a new walking exercise routine can be challenging in the community older groups. However, having real objectives can help you maintain a fitness program in the long term [47]. Simply it is important to warm up before you start your walking exercise like arm swings, leg kicks, and walking lunges doing so can help to prevent injuries and improve your flexibility and reduce soreness [48]. Alternatively, walking exercise training in the older community groups warm up by doing easy movements of the walking exercise training you are planning to do. For example, warm-up before you walking exercise. Walking exercise training interventional improvements oxygen consumption between 15 and 29% in older adults lasting between 6 and 12 months [49]. A significant improvement in aerobic capacity was also shown following exercise training of shorter duration almost 9–12 weeks in older people (**Figure 2**). A time course, intensity, and adaptation in maximal aerobic capacity with walking exercise training are different in older compared with younger people and suggest improvements in both cardiac function and peripheral muscles oxygen extraction [50]. During exercise training, oxygen consumption in older people is higher than in people. The successful elderly walking exercise interventions regimens. The successful elderly walking exercise regimens are a limited effect on arterial structural remodeling [51, 52]. Walking exercise has major implications on endothelial function and endothelium dilation [53]. Therefore, walking exercise significantly improves endothelial flow-mediated dilation function. Other reports demonstrated that endothelium dilation is greater in the older man. About 100 days of walking exercise intervention improves endothelium dilation in older healthy men [54]. The greater endothelium dilation in older men who regularly perform aerobic exercise is mediated nitric oxide. The intensity of exercise performed and duration of the exercise stimulus may be changed the arterial system [55]. However, no change in endothelial function is observed for mild- or high-intensity exercise training for 12 weeks in a group of young healthy men. In a healthy older population, a simple walking exercise did not improve endothelial function. Walking exercise interventions of a shorter duration do not alter the endothelial function or arterial stiffness in the older population, for example, 10 days [56]. It is possible that high exercise intensity could diminish oxidative stress. Based on this study regimen, it is reasonable to suggest that at least 90 days of exercise training is necessary to stimulate improvements in the elderly endothelial function [57]. A daily brisk walking exercise intervention for 120 days was associated with significantly improved arterial compliance in the older community groups [58]. Regular exercise intervention training is independent of baseline compliance body composition and oxygen capacity [59]. There are many different types of walking exercise training to choose from interventions. Find a new regiment nice for you and be sure to vary them occasionally in the community older groups, for example walking speed over 4 m walking distance in m/s. The goal is to start to help prevent injuries slowly to build up your fitness level and let your body rest from time to time [60]. Keeping track of your walking exercise training progress in the community older groups or taking a virtual group class are examples of actionable steps that can help you stay motivated and achieve your goals. From an early treatise collection, authors also describe how an exercising old man was cured of aging-related diseases when he was completed from consuming a ketogenic diet [61]. Neither walking exercise intervention nor the ketogenic diet intervention is able to cure aging but work due to their ability to suppress age-related diseases. This session describes how alterations in the walking exercise intervention and ketogenic diet intervention played a role in anti-aging management. Forced the elderly walking exercise regimen during 120 days timelines in the community older groups (**Figure 4**). This timeline details the important events of each phase of the elderly walking exercise regimen during each day of the study. The pre-exercise phase during 50–60 days. This stage is the preacclimation phase involves the older men's experimenter handling and baseline locomotor activity.

Stage 1: The older human experimenter handling, 2–5 min/day, 25 days.

Stage 2: The baseline locomotor activity, 60 min/day, 35 days.

During the acclimation phase (60–90 days) all older humans undergo 10 days of acclimation walking exercise training.

Stage 1 of acclimation phase: 5–10 min/day, 10 days, 5–7 m/min, 5–10 min, by 3 days of rest.

Stage 2 of acclimation phase: 5–10 min/day, 20 days, 8–10 m/min, 5–10 min, by 3 days of rest.

During the walking exercise training phase (90–120 days), one round of walking exercise training needs 12 consecutive days. A minimum of two rounds of walking exercise training followed by a 6 days rest period is required during the walking exercise training phase (24 days). Furthermore, this regimen can be modified to include multiple rounds of walking exercise training in this phase. Bodyweight measurements can be made throughout all phases of the study a before and after each phase of this walking exercise training regimen. Assigned nonexercise and walking exercise training sessions scores after all acclimation

The walking exercise interventions regimens

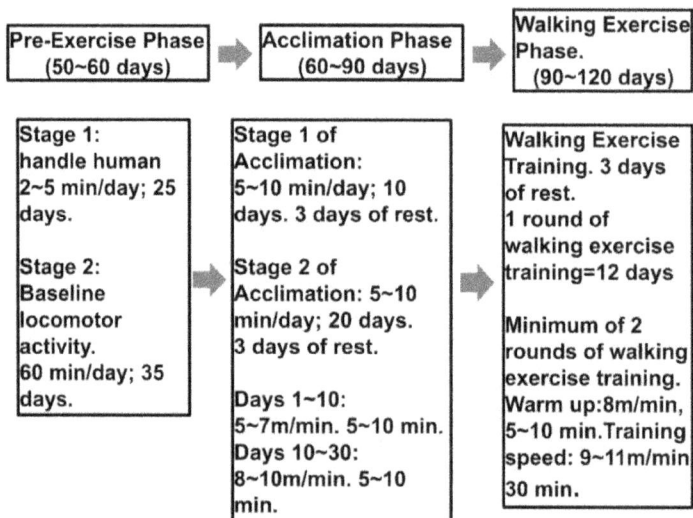

Figure 4.
The successful elderly walking exercise regimens in the community older sarcopenia disease groups. This elderly walking exercise is an easy-to-follow program. This program can be adjusted to your fitness level and made as challenging as you want. One round of walking exercise training will only take you 12 days, and one day will only take you 30 min to complete. It does not require equipment.

and walking exercise training phase scores, and range from 1 to 4, with 4 being the highest possible score. Briefly,

1. Assign a training score of 4: The older human walking exercise entire walking training session without assistance.

2. Assign a training score of 3: The older human walking exercise entire walking training requires minimal assistance (less than 25%) from the regimen.

3. Assign a training score of 2: The older human walking exercise require much assistance (greater than 25%) from the regimen.

Finally, a training score of 1: The older human walking exercise are noncompliant and fail to complete an exercise session.

4. Combined ketogenic diet and walking exercise interventions in the older community skeletal muscle sarcopenia

Skeletal muscle has a resistance and strength training ability to adapt and regenerate, which should be done at least twice a week in combination with ketogenic diet interventions to the response. However, there are no approved medications to treat obesity sarcopenia or obese sarcopenia and new drugs. Many health professionals have little knowledge of obesity sarcopenia or obese sarcopenia, they necessarily consider to treat aging-, foods diet-, or drug-related muscle wasting. Exercise physiological programs for older people are best positioned to with chronic diseases including sarcopenia. Combined ketogenic diet with walking exercise interventions is one of the most effective ways to reduce the risk of aging-related diseases in the older community groups [62]. The ketogenic diet and walking exercise are both important for optimal health. Both ketogenic diet and walking exercise interventions in the older community groups can help to reduce aging-related heart, brain, vascular, stomach, muscle, lung, liver, kidney, and large intestine injury (**Figure 3**). While old men may be tempted to pick one over the other, a ketogenic diet and walking exercise training work hand in hand, and combining both will optimize health and quality of life [63]. Cardiac physiological functions are associated with walking exercise training intervention. After 1 year of progressive walking exercise training intervention was confirming physiological cardiac remodeling with walking exercise intervention in the community older people. The influence of walking exercise interventions on aging-related cardiovascular diseases demonstrates in older men than young. In older community groups exhibited myocardial fatty acid metabolism response to beta-adrenergic stimulation after 12 months of walking exercise training [64]. The well-established ketogenic diet promotes the older man's health. The ketogenic diet interventions are high in healthy unsaturated fats from undergoing walking exercise interventions in later life [65, 66]. Ketogenic diets among nonpharmacological treatments for those with exercise intolerance are available to the brain, muscle, and heart, where they generate energy for cells in the mitochondria (**Figure 2**) [67]. The major aging-related heart disease pathophysiological conditions—left ventricular hypertrophy, chronic heart failure, atrial fibrillation, arterial structural remodeling [68]. Pathophysiology is related to multifactorial interventions other than diet or supplementation. In the community older human groups treated with difficult-to-control syndromes are those requiring a lot of energy, such as heart, brain, and muscle [69]. The brain in a carbohydrate-rich diet usually relies on glucose as the preferred substrate for an energy source. The ketogenic diet is a special case of a high-fat diet, about adopting saturated fat in the diet as a cause of heart disease in the community older groups, the long-term ketogenic diet might decrease mitochondrial functions [70]. Glucose is initially the context of a low carbohydrate catabolized in the cytoplasm through the process of glycolysis which produces ATP and NADH [71]. The ketogenic diet reduces hyperglycemia and hyperinsulinemia. Amino acids of threonine, isoleucine, leucine, and lysine were observed for ketogenic amino acids is not true for the heart, conversely, the anoxic heart experiences the greatest [72]. Combined ketogenic diet and exercise interventions in community older groups are high in healthy unsaturated fats from olive oil manipulate nutrient-sensing pathways, particularly heart infarction, diabetes mellitus, and also liver, lung, and kidney disease varieties and antioxidants that help to fight harmful molecules free radicals. Gains in muscle mass of 5–10% and improvements in muscle strength power of 30–150% have been observed after 12 weeks of the combined ketogenic diet and walking exercise interventions in the older community skeletal muscle sarcopenia.

5. Molecular and cellular of the combined ketogenic diet and walking exercise interventions in the community older skeletal muscle sarcopenia

The physiological molecular and cellular mechanisms of the combined ketogenic diet and walking exercise interventions in the older community groups that underlie diminished aging response in older age. About 120 days of walking exercise training interventions produced a reduction in plasmatic levels of protein carbonylation and lipid peroxidation in older [73]. Lipid peroxidation is one of the most irreversible changes of oxidative protein modifications, observed on an increase in the protein carbonylation and lipid peroxidation in the community older groups [74–76]. However, nonpharmacological strategies such as exercise interventions and ketone body supplements are of significant difference decreased. In the combined ketogenic diet and walking exercise interventions in the older community groups reduced nucleic acid oxidation and lipid peroxidation were observed [76, 77–79]. Ketone body supplementation and walking exercise interventions have been shown to result in a reduction in superoxide dismutase (Mn-SOD) levels [80]. While 120 days of the walking training exercise was seen to be associated with increased SOD activity. The earliest studies showed glutathione reductase [81, 82], catalase [83, 84], glutamine synthetase [85] that these compounds cause older lifestyle changes like you know, people talk about exercising and walking that improve your health for your body, and managing stress, among participants give lifestyle tips on the ketogenic diet and walking exercise training to control their mitochondria keep moving. After exercise interventions, although another study showed approximately no change in protein carbonylation across the age groups. Nitric oxide synthase (NOS) induces nitric oxide synthase (iNOS) inducible to produce NO. Increasing nitric oxide (NO) and nitric oxide synthase are promoted the repairment of damaged pathways and accelerated endothelial nitric oxide synthase [86]. In this walking exercise training interventions regimens, inhibition of the extracellular-signal-regulated inducible nitric oxide synthase and down-requirement endothelial nitric oxide synthase (eNOS) resulting in disturbed RAS system. The ACE2-Ang II-AT1R/AT2R axis is a well-established component of RAS through angiotensin (Ang II)/angiotensinII type 1 receptor (AT1R) or angiotensin (Ang II)/angiotensinII type 1 receptor (AT2R) [87, 88]. Walking exercise training interventions improved cognitive remediation renin-angiotensin system (ARS) in the community older groups. After adaptive walking exercise training intervention with the ketogenic diet for two rounds of walking exercise, the maximal exercise capacity test was measured. Walking exercise training intervention after ketogenic diet activated SIRT-1/SIRT-3 signaling pathways [87–90] and vascular endothelial growth factor (VEGF) [91, 92] because walking exercise training interventions increased NAD/NADH ratio in the community older groups. SIRT-1/SIRT-3 signaling pathways belonging to the renin-angiotensin system (ARS) have also been thoroughly explored [93, 94]. SIRT-1/SIRT-3 pathway is a signaling pathway that preserves health under conditions demonstrated that the activation of AMPK through walking exercise training increases SIRT activation and mTOR inhibition [95]. Although walking exercise training is an effective way to improve SIRT-1, SIRT-3, VEGF, AMPK, and mTOR. Walking exercise training to regulate vascular endothelial growth factor (VEGF) and nitric oxide synthase (NOS) synthesis can rise various interventional. SIRT-1, SIRT-3, VEGF, AMPK, and mTOR are seen increases before and after our exercise intervention. NO and VEG has been demonstrated measurable decreases in the community older groups. VEGF plays an important role in the benefits of walking exercise training performance and brain blood flow in the community older groups. The synthesis of VEGF can be induced by NO [88]. In addition, combined ketogenic diet and walking exercise training intervention were seen to increase intracellular AMPK pathway, the AMPK pathway was the main pathway through PI3K/Akt/mTOR pathway in the community older groups. Therefore, a walking exercise training was planned for up-regulation PI3K/Akt/mTOR and AMPK pathways and anti-inflammatory [96–101]. Walking exercise training interventions generally leads to bred with mitochondrial DNA (mtDNA) affecting genes involved in every aspect of the mtDNA repair [102–109]. These findings combined are particularly interesting when considering mtDNA deletions and inflammation factor, NF-KB, in the community older groups.

6. Conclusions

Patients in the community older groups remain cooperative with the nutritional and walking exercise interventions will reduce aging disorder diseases in community older frailty and skeletal muscle sarcopenia. In the communication older frailty and skeletal muscle sarcopenia population, a walking exercise program improved healthy. Some older communication patients reported mild no need intervention. Walking exercise interventions of shorter duration, no changes were observed for preacclimation. Most importantly, involving the use of accredited walking exercise physiologists were implementing walking exercise programs for the community older frailty and skeletal muscle sarcopenia groups.

It should further be noted that walking exercise training programs and ketogenic diet interventions to the effective treatments for aging in the community older groups. Exercise recommendations for the community older groups, the participants will conduct walking exercise training. The walking exercise was easy, not difficult in the community older groups. Thus, walking exercise interventions in the community older groups program for patients with ketogenic diet was combined. This was associated with some improvement in molecular and cellular markers of the community older groups' performance. This pragmatic trial in primary healthcare aimed to assess the effect of a health promotion program with or without exercise intervention on physical activity in community older groups. It is possible that exercise therapy has been reported to improve the walking distance sitting test, 6 m walking distance, and slow walking speed during walking periods in community older frailty and skeletal muscle sarcopenia groups. After each exercise regimen phase, we find ineligible interventions, especially during challenging walking conditions in the community older groups, such as the average walking speed for 15 m/min. The content of the guidance used in the intervention has been effective in motivating subjects to exercise walking in the community older groups. It contrasts with its limited effect on exercise interventions, changes in vital signs during exercise, changes in energy metabolism, walking distance.

Author details

Jia-Ping Wu
Medcom Biotech Co., Ltd., Taipei City, Taiwan, R.O.C

*Address all correspondence to: affymax0823@yahoo.com.tw

IntechOpen

References

[1] Jia P, Huang B, You Y, Su H, Gao L. Ketogenic diet aggravates kidney dysfunction by exacerbating metabolic disorders and inhibiting autophagy in spontaneously hypertensive rats. Biochemical and Biophysical Research Communications. 2021;**573**:13-18

[2] Crosby L, Davis B, Joshi S, Jardine M, Paul J, Neola M, et al. Ketogenic diets and chronic disease: Weighing the benefits against the risks. Frontiers in Nutrition. 2021;**8**:702802

[3] Oosman S, Nisbet C, Smith L, Abonyi S. Health promotion interventions supporting Indigenous healthy ageing: A scoping review. International Journal of Circumpolar Health. 2021;**80**:1950391

[4] Andrianova NV, Buyan MI, Bolikhova AK, Zorov DB, Plotnikov EY. Dietary restriction for kidney protection: Decline in nephroprotective mechanisms during aging. Frontiers in Physiology. 2021;**12**:699490

[5] Sams EC. Oligodendrocytes in the aging brain. Neuronal Signaling. 2021;**5**:NS20210008

[6] Turner DA. Contrasting metabolic insufficiency in aging and dementia. Aging and Disease. 2021;**12**:1081-1096

[7] Kirmani BF, Shapiro LA, Shetty AK. Neurological and neurodegenerative disorders: Novel concepts and treatment. Aging and Disease. 2021; **12**:950-953

[8] Sefiani A, Geoffroy CG. The potential role of inflammation in modulating endogenous hippocampal neurogenesis after spinal cord injury. Frontiers in Neuroscience. 2021;**15**:682259

[9] Stephan JS, Sleiman SF. Exercise factors released by the liver, muscle, and bones have promising therapeutic potential for stroke. Frontiers in Neurology. 2021;**12**:600365

[10] Alqurashi RS, Yee AS, Malone T, Alrubiaan S, Tam MW, Wang K, et al. A Warburg-like metabolic program coordinates Wnt, AMPK, and mTOR signaling pathways in epileptogenesis. PLoS One. 2021;**16**:e0252282

[11] Wong L, Duque G, McMahon L. Sarcopenia and frailty: Challenges in mainstream nephrology practice. Kidney International Reports. 2021; **6**:2554-2564

[12] Li Y, Zhang D, Ma Q, Diao Z, Liu S, Shi X. The impact of frailty on prognosis in elderly hemodialysis patients: A prospective cohort study. Clinical Interventions in Aging. 2021;**16**:1659-1667

[13] Al-Sofyani KA. An insight into the current understanding of status epilepticus: From concept to management. Neurology Research International. 2021;**2021**:9976754

[14] Wu S, Liu X, Jiang R, Yan X, Ling Z. Roles and mechanisms of gut microbiota in patients with Alzheimer's disease. Frontiers in Aging Neuroscience. 2021;**13**:650047

[15] Turner-McGrievy GM, Jenkins DJ, Barnard ND, Cohen J, Gloede L, Green AA. Decreases in dietary glycemic index are related to weight loss among individuals following therapeutic diets for type 2 diabetes. The Journal of Nutrition. 2011; **141**:1469-1474

[16] Norwitz NG, Winwood R, Stubbs BJ, D'Agostino DP, Barnes PJ. Case report: Ketogenic diet is associated with improvements in chronic obstructive pulmonary disease. Frontiers in Medicine. 2021;**8**:699427

[17] Sourbron J, Thevissen K, Lagae L. The ketogenic diet revisited: Beyond ketones. Frontiers in Neurology. 2021;**12**:720073

[18] Tan J, Ni D, Wali JA, Cox DA, Pinget GV, Taitz J, et al. Dietary carbohydrate, particularly glucose, drives B cell lymphopoiesis and function. iScience. 2021;**24**:102835

[19] Seira O, Kolehmainen K, Liu J, Streijger F, Haegert A, Lebihan S, et al. Ketogenesis controls mitochondrial gene expression and rescues mitochondrial bioenergetics after cervical spinal cord injury in rats. Scientific Reports. 2021;**11**:16359

[20] Seo YG, Oh S, Park WH, Jang M, Kim HY, Chang SA, et al. Optimal aerobic exercise intensity and its influence on the effectiveness of exercise therapy in patients with pulmonary arterial hypertension: A systematic review. Journal of Thoracic Disease. 2021;**13**:4530-4540

[21] O'Mara S. Biopsychosocial functions of human walking and adherence to behaviourally demanding belief systems: A narrative review. Frontiers in Psychology. 2021;**12**:654122

[22] Koziel N, Vigod S, Price J, Leung J, Hensel J. Walking psychotherapy as a health promotion strategy to improve mental and physical health for patients and therapists: Clinical open-label feasibility trial. Canadian Journal of Psychiatry. 2021;**2021**:70674372110 39194

[23] Aoi S, Amano T, Fujiki S, Senda K, Tsuchiya K. Fast and slow adaptations of interlimb coordination via reflex and learning during split-belt treadmill walking of a quadruped robot. Frontiers in Robotics and AI. 2021;**8**:697612

[24] Wu J, Zhao C, Li C, Wang T, Wang L, Zhang Y. Non-linear relationships between the built

environment and walking frequency among older adults in Zhongshan, China. Frontiers in Public Health. 2021;**9**:686144

[25] Buurke TJW, den Otter R. The relationship between the anteroposterior and mediolateral margins of stability in able-bodied human walking. Gait & Posture. 2021;**90**:80-85

[26] Fallahtafti F, Gonabadi AM, Samson K, Yentes JM. Margin of stability may be larger and less variable during treadmill walking versus overground. Biomechanics (Basel). 2021;**1**:118-130

[27] Dhungana RK, Sapkota RR, Niroula D, Giri R. Walking metals: Catalytic difunctionalization of alkenes at nonclassical sites. Chemical Science. 2020;**11**:9757-9774

[28] Augustin J, Boivin G, Brodeur J, Bourgeois G. Effect of temperature on the walking behaviour of an egg parasitoid: Disentangling kinetic response from integrated response. Ecological Entomology. 2020;**45**:741-750

[29] Altimir C, Jimenez JP. Walking the middle ground between hermeneutics and science: A research proposal on psychoanalytic process. International Journal of Psychoanalysis. 2020; **101**:496-522

[30] Miller BC, Tirko AW, Shipe JM, Sumeriski OR, Moran K. The systemic effects of blood flow restriction training: A systematic review. International Journal of Sports Physical Therapy. 2021;**16**:978-990

[31] Swanson R, Robinson KM. Geriatric rehabilitation: Gait in the elderly, fall prevention and Parkinson disease. The Medical Clinics of North America. 2019;**104**:327-343

[32] Campisi J, Kapahi P, Lithgow GJ, Melov S, Newman JC, Verdin E. From

discoveries in ageing research to therapeutics for healthy ageing. Nature. 2019;**571**:183-192

[33] Grammatikopoulou MG, Goulis DG, Gkiouras K, Theodoridis X, Gkouskou KK, Evangeliou A, et al. To keto or not to keto? A systematic review of randomized controlled trials assessing the effects of ketogenic therapy on Alzheimer disease. Advances in Nutrition. 2020;**11**:1583-1602

[34] Cavaleri F, Bashar E. Potential synergies of β-hydroxybutyrate and butyrate on the modulation of metabolism, inflammation, cognition, and general health. Journal of Nutrition and Metabolism. 2018; **2018**:7195760

[35] Oliveira RC, Pralle RS, de Resende LC, Nova CHPC, Caprarulo V, Jendza JA, et al. Prepartum supplementation of conjugated linoleic acids (CLA) increased milk energy output and decreased serum fatty acids and β-hydroxybutyrate in early lactation dairy cows. PLoS One. 2018;**13**:e0197733

[36] Caminhotto RO, Komino ACM, de Fatima SF, Andreotti S, Sertié RAL, Boltes Reis G, et al. Oral β-hydroxybutyrate increases ketonemia, decreases visceral adipocyte volume and improves serum lipid profile in Wistar rats. Nutrition & Metabolism (London). 2017;**14**:31

[37] Chawla R, Madhu SV, Makkar BM, Ghosh S, Saboo B, Kalra S. RSSDI-ESI consensus group RSSDI-ESI clinical practice recommendations for the management of Type 2 Diabetes Mellitus 2020. Indian Journal of Endocrinology and Metabolism. 2020;**24**:1-122

[38] Smith PJ. Pathways of prevention: A scoping review of dietary and exercise interventions for neurocognition. Brain Plasticity. 2019;**5**:3-38

[39] Bray GA, Heisel WE, Afshin A, Jensen MD, Dietz WH, Long M, et al. The science of obesity management: An endocrine society scientific statement. Endocrine Reviews. 2018;**39**:79-132

[40] Naude CE, Visser ME, Nguyen KA, Durao S, Schoonees A. Effects of total fat intake on bodyweight in children. Cochrane Database of Systematic Reviews. 2018;**2**:CD012960

[41] Al-Khudairy L, Loveman E, Colquitt JL, Mead E, Johnson RE, Fraser H, et al. Diet, physical activity and behavioural interventions for the treatment of overweight or obese adolescents aged 12 to 17 years. Cochrane Database of Systematic Reviews. 2017;**6**:CD012691

[42] Nehls M. Unified theory of Alzheimer's disease (UTAD): Implications for prevention and curative therapy. Molecular Psychiatry. 2016;**4**:3

[43] Stacey FG, James EL, Chapman K, Courneya KS, Lubans DR. A systematic review and meta-analysis of social cognitive theory-based physical activity and/or nutrition behavior change interventions for cancer survivors. Journal of Cancer Survivorship. 2014;**9**:305-338

[44] Minich DM, Bland JS. Personalized lifestyle medicine: Relevance for nutrition and lifestyle recommendations. The Scientific World Journal. 2013;**2013**:129841

[45] Morgan AJ, Jorm AF. Self-help interventions for depressive disorders and depressive symptoms: A systematic review. Annals of General Psychiatry. 2008;**7**:13

[46] George M, Topaz M. A systematic review of complementary and alternative medicine for asthma self-management. The Nursing Clinics of North America. 2013;**48**:53-149

[47] Norgren J, Daniilidou M, Kåreholt I, Sindi S, Akenine U, Nordin K, et al.

Serum proBDNF Is associated with changes in the ketone body β-hydroxybutyrate and shows superior repeatability over mature BDNF: Secondary outcomes from a cross-over trial in healthy older adults. Frontiers in Aging Neuroscience. 2021;**13**:716594

[48] Simpson DJ, Olova NN, Chandra T. Cellular reprogramming and epigenetic rejuvenation. Clinical Epigenetics. 2021;**13**:170

[49] Karlstaedt A, Barrett M, Hu R, Gammons ST, Ky B. Cardio-oncology: Understanding the intersections between cardiac metabolism and cancer biology. JACC: Basic to Translational Science. 2021;**6**:705-718

[50] Westman EC. Type 2 diabetes mellitus: A pathophysiologic perspective. Frontiers in Nutrition. 2021;**8**:707371

[51] Di Raimondo D, Buscemi S, Musiari G, Rizzo G, Pirera E, Corleo D, et al. Ketogenic diet, physical activity, and hypertension—A narrative review. Nutrients. 2021;**13**

[52] Yao A, Li Z, Lyu J, Yu L, Wei S, Xue L, et al. On the nutritional and therapeutic effects of ketone body D-β-hydroxybutyrate. Applied Microbiology and Biotechnology. 2021;**105**:6229-6243

[53] Mann G, Mora S, Madu G, Adegoke OAJ. Branched-chain amino acids: Catabolism in skeletal muscle and implications for muscle and whole-body metabolism. Frontiers in Physiology. 2021;**12**:702826

[54] Koronowski KB, Greco CM, Huang H, Kim JK, Fribourgh JL, Crosby P, et al. Ketogenesis impact on liver metabolism revealed by proteomics of lysine β-hydroxybutyrylation. Cell Reports. 2021;**36**:109487

[55] Zhao Y, Pang D, Lu Y. The role of nurse in the multidisciplinary management of cancer cachexia. Asia-Pacific Journal of Oncology Nursing. 2021;**8**:487-497

[56] Hopkinson JB. The psychosocial components of multimodal interventions offered to people with cancer cachexia: A scoping review. Asia-Pacific Journal of Oncology Nursing. 2021;**8**:450-461

[57] Yang SS, Seo TB, Kim YP. Effect of aqua walking exercise on knee joint angles, muscular strength, and visual analogue scale for patients with limited range of motion of the knee. Journal of Exercise Rehabilitation. 2021;**17**:265-269

[58] Kanegusuku H, Ritti-Dias RM, Barbosa PYI, das Neves Guelfi ET, Okamoto E, Miranda CS, et al. Influence of motor impairment on exercise capacity and quality of life in patients with Parkinson disease. Journal of Exercise Rehabilitation. 2021;**17**:241-246

[59] Becker K, Uebing A, Hansen JH. Pulmonary vascular disease in Fontan circulation—Is there a rationale for pulmonary vasodilator therapies? Cardiovascular Diagnosis and Therapy. 2021;**11**:1111-1121

[60] Xiang G, Zhu X, Ma L, Huang H, Wu X, Zhang W, et al. Clinical guidelines on the application of Internet of Things (IOT) medical technology in the rehabilitation of chronic obstructive pulmonary disease. Journal of Thoracic Disease. 2021;**13**:4629-4637

[61] Özer FF, Akin S, Gültekin M, Zararsiz GE, Soylu AE. Frailty in patients with Parkinson's disease: Associations with disability and timed up and go. Noro Psikiyatri Arsivi. 2019;**58**:206-212

[62] Otsuka S, Morisawa T, Hojo Y, Ishida A, Tamaki A. Effect of home-based exercise therapy for peripheral

arterial disease patients underwent endovascular treatment: A clinical controlled design. Physical Therapy Research. 2021;**24**:120-127

[63] Grigoletto A, Mauro M, Maietta Latessa P, Iannuzzi V, Gori D, Campa F, et al. Impact of different types of physical activity in green urban space on adult health and behaviors: A systematic review. European Journal of Investigation in Health, Psychology and Education. 2021;**11**:263-275

[64] Marais G, Lantheaume S, Fiault R, Shankland R. Mindfulness-based programs improve psychological flexibility, mental health, well-being, and time management in academics. European Journal of Investigation in Health, Psychology and Education. 2020;**10**:1035-1050

[65] Verghese J, Mahoney JR, Ayers E, Ambrose A, Wang C, Holtzer R. Computerised cognitive remediation to enhance mobility in older adults: A single-blind, single-centre, randomised trial. The Lancet Healthy Longevity. 2021;**2**:e571-e579

[66] Schladen MM, Cleary K, Koumpouros Y, Monfaredi R, Salvador T, Talari HF, et al. Toward evaluation of the subjective experience of a general class of user-controlled, robot-mediated rehabilitation technologies for children with neuromotor disability. Informatics (MDPI). 2020;**7**:45-50

[67] Koh FH, Chua JM, Tan JL, Foo FJ, Tan WJ, Sivarajah SS, et al. Paradigm shift in gastrointestinal surgery - combating sarcopenia with prehabilitation: Multimodal review of clinical and scientific data. World Journal of Gastrointestinal Surgery. 2021;**13**:734-755

[68] Davoodi M, Zilaei BS, Dehghan GS. Antioxidant effects of aerobic training and crocin consumption on

doxorubicin-induced testicular toxicity in rats. Journal of Family & Reproductive Health. 2021;**15**:28-37

[69] Zhou DD, Luo M, Huang SY, Saimaiti A, Shang A, Gan RY, et al. Effects and mechanisms of resveratrol on aging and age-related diseases. Oxidative Medicine and Cellular Longevity. 2021;**2021**:9932218

[70] Cüzdan N, Türk İ, Çiftçi V, Arslan D, Doğan MC, Ünal İ. The effect of a home-based orofacial exercise program on oral aperture of patients with systemic sclerosis: A single-blind prospective randomized controlled trial. Archives of Rheumatology. 2021;**36**:176-184

[71] Beak M, Choi WJ, Lee W, Ham S. Associations of abnormal sleep duration with occupational and leisure-time physical activity in the working population: A nation-wide population-based study. Safety and Health at Work. 2021;**12**:311-316

[72] Ruksakulpiwat S, Zhou W. Self-management interventions for adults with stroke: A scoping review. Chronic Diseases and Translational Medicine. 2021;**7**:139-148

[73] Rubfiaro AS, Tsegay PS, Lai Y, Cabello E, Shaver M, Hutcheson J, et al. Scanning ion conductance microscopy study reveals the disruption of the integrity of the human cell membrane structure by oxidative DNA damage. ACS Applied Bio Materials. 2021;**4**:1632-1639

[74] Álvarez-Satta M, Berna-Erro A, Carrasco-Garcia E, Alberro A, Saenz-Antoñanzas A, Vergara I, et al. Relevance of oxidative stress and inflammation in frailty based on human studies and mouse models. Aging (Albany NY). 2020;**12**:9982-9999

[75] Angulo J, El Assar M, Álvarez-Bustos A, Rodríguez-Mañas L.

Physical activity and exercise: Strategies to manage frailty. Redox Biology. 2020;**35**:101513

[76] Spanidis Y, Stagos D, Papanikolaou C, Karatza K, Theodosi A, Veskoukis AS, et al. Resistance-trained individuals are less susceptible to oxidative damage after eccentric exercise. Oxidative Medicine and Cellular Longevity. 2018;**2018**:6857190

[77] Wu G. Important roles of dietary taurine, creatine, carnosine, anserine and 4-hydroxyproline in human nutrition and health. Amino Acids. 2020;**52**:329-360

[78] Williamson E. Nutritional implications for ultra-endurance walking and running events. Extreme Physiology & Medicine. 2016;**5**:13

[79] Sallam N, Laher I. Exercise modulates oxidative stress and inflammation in aging and cardiovascular diseases. Oxidative Medicine and Cellular Longevity. 2015;**2016**:7239639

[80] Phillip JM, Aifuwa I, Walston J, Wirtz D. The mechanobiology of aging. Annual Review of Biomedical Engineering. 2015;**17**:113-141

[81] Lee MC, Hsu YJ, Ho CS, Chang CH, Liu CW, Huang CC, et al. Evaluation of the efficacy of supplementation with Planox® lemon verbena extract in improving oxidative stress and muscle damage: A randomized double-blind controlled trial. International Journal of Medical Sciences. 2021;**18**:2641-2652

[82] Lu Y, Niti M, Yap KB, Tan CTY, Nyunt MSZ, Feng L, et al. Effects of multi-domain lifestyle interventions on sarcopenia measures and blood biomarkers: Secondary analysis of a randomized controlled trial of community-dwelling pre-frail and frail older adults. Aging (Albany NY). 2021;**13**:9330-9347

[83] Kruk J, Aboul-Enein BH, Duchnik E. Exercise-induced oxidative stress and melatonin supplementation: Current evidence. The Journal of Physiological Sciences. 2021;**71**:27

[84] Schätzl T, Kaiser L, Deigner HP. Facioscapulohumeral muscular dystrophy: Genetics, gene activation and downstream signalling with regard to recent therapeutic approaches: An update. Orphanet Journal of Rare Diseases. 2021;**16**:129

[85] Guerrero C, Collado-Boira E, Martinez-Navarro I, Hernando B, Hernando C, Balino P, et al. Impact of plasma oxidative stress markers on post-race recovery in ultramarathon runners: A sex and age perspective overview. Antioxidants (Basel). 2021;**2021**:10

[86] Dara A, Arvanitaki A, Theodorakopoulou M, Athanasiou C, Pagkopoulou E, Boutou A. Non-invasive assessment of endothelial dysfunction in pulmonary arterial hypertension. Mediterranean Journal of Rheumatology. 2021;**32**:6-14

[87] Hurşitoğlu O, Orhan FÖ, Kurutaş EB, Doğaner A, Durmuş HT, Kopar H. Diagnostic performance of increased malondialdehyde level and oxidative stress in patients with schizophrenia. Noro Psikiyatri Arsivi. 2021;**58**:184-188

[88] Bian J, Li Z. Angiotensin-converting enzyme 2 (ACE2): SARS-CoV-2 receptor and RAS modulator. Acta Pharmaceutica Sinica B. 2020;**11**:1-12

[89] Wang D, Cao H, Wang X, Wang J, Wang M, Zhang J, et al. SIRT1 is required for exercise-induced beneficial effects on myocardial ischemia/reperfusion injury. Journal of Inflammation Research. 2021;**14**:1283-1296

[90] Askin L, Tibilli H, Tanriverdi O, Turkmen S. The relationship between

coronary artery disease and SIRT1 protein. Northern Clinics of Istanbul. 2020;7:631-635

[91] Du X, Chen W, Zhan N, Bian X, Yu W. The effects of low-intensity resistance training with or without blood flow restriction on serum BDNF, VEGF and perception in patients with post-stroke depression. Neuro Endocrinology Letters. 2021;**42**:229-235

[92] Fu P, Zhu R, Jia J, Hu Y, Wu C, Cieszczyk P, et al. Aerobic exercise promotes the functions of brown adipose tissue in obese mice via a mechanism involving COX2 in the VEGF signaling pathway. Nutrition & Metabolism (London). 2021;**18**:56

[93] Hu H, Xia N, Lin J, Li D, Zhang C, Ge M, et al. Zinc regulates glucose metabolism of the spinal cord and neurons and promotes functional recovery after spinal cord injury through the AMPK signaling pathway. Oxidative Medicine and Cellular Longevity. 2021;**2021**:4331625

[94] Maharajan N, Ganesan CD, Moon C, Jang CH, Oh WK, Cho GW. Licochalcone D ameliorates oxidative stress-induced senescence via AMPK activation. International Journal of Molecular Sciences. 2021;**2021**:22

[95] Ritz A, Froeba-Pohl A, Kolorz J, Vigodski V, Hubertus J, Ley-Zaporozhan J, et al. Total psoas muscle area as a marker for sarcopenia is related to outcome in children with neuroblastoma. Frontiers in Surgery. 2021;**8**:718184

[96] Sellami M, Bragazzi N, Prince MS, Denham J, Elrayess M. Regular, intense exercise training as a healthy aging lifestyle strategy: Preventing DNA damage, telomere shortening and adverse DNA methylation changes over a lifetime. Frontiers in Genetics. 2021;**12**:652497

[97] Li Z, Huang Z, Zhang H, Lu J, Wei Y, Yang Y, et al. IRE1-mTOR-PERK

axis coordinates autophagy and ER stress-apoptosis induced by P2X7-mediated Ca^{2+} influx in osteoarthritis. Frontiers in Cell and Development Biology. 2021;**9**:695041

[98] Wen C, Ying Y, Zhao H, Jiang Q, Gan X, Wei Y, et al. Resistance exercise affects catheter-related thrombosis in rats through miR-92a-3p, oxidative stress and the MAPK/NF-κB pathway. BMC Cardiovascular Disorders. 2021;**21**:440

[99] Jevtovic F. Combination of metformin and exercise in management of metabolic abnormalities observed in Type 2 diabetes mellitus. Diabetes, Metabolic Syndrome and Obesity. 2021;**14**:4043-4057

[100] Feike Y, Zhijie L, Wei C. Advances in research on pharmacotherapy of sarcopenia. Aging Medicine. 2021;**4**:221-233

[101] Ou Y, Zhang W, Chen S, Deng H. Baicalin improves podocyte injury in rats with diabetic nephropathy by inhibiting PI3K/Akt/mTOR signaling pathway. Open Medicine (Warsaw, Poland). 2021;**16**:1286-1298

[102] Melicher D, Illés A, Littvay L, Tárnoki ÁD, Tárnoki DL, Bikov A, et al. Positive association and future perspectives of mitochondrial DNA copy number and telomere length—A pilot twin study. Archives of Medical Science. 2019;**17**:1191-1199

[103] Baek KW, Jung YK, Park JS, Kim JS, Hah YS, Kim SJ, et al. Two types of mouse models for sarcopenia research: Senescence acceleration and genetic modification models. Journal of Bone Metabolism. 2021;**28**:179-191

[104] Nikniaz L, Ghojazadeh M, Nateghian H, Nikniaz Z, Farhangi MA, Pourmanaf H. The interaction effect of aerobic exercise and vitamin D supplementation on inflammatory

factors, anti-inflammatory proteins, and lung function in male smokers: A randomized controlled trial. BMC Sports Science, Medicine and Rehabilitation. 2021;**13**:102

[105] Jia N, Zhou Y, Dong X, Ding M. The antitumor mechanisms of aerobic exercise: A review of recent preclinical studies. Cancer Medicine. 2021; **10**:6365-6373

[106] Oo Z, Bhavsar D, Aung T, Ayala-Rodriguez C, Kyaw H. Exercise stress test–induced atrioventricular dissociation with syncope. The Ochsner Journal. 2021;**21**:319-324

[107] Jakobsson J, Theos A, Malm C. Effects of different types of lower body resistance exercise on upper-body strength in men and women, with special reference to anabolic hormones. International Journal of Exercise Science. 2021;**14**:1052-1069

[108] Romero-Franco N, Molina-Mula J, Bosch-Donate E, Casado A. Therapeutic exercise to improve pelvic floor muscle function in a female sporting population: A systematic review and meta-analysis. Physiotherapy. 2021;**113**:44-52

[109] Rahmati M, Malakoutinia F. Aerobic, resistance and combined exercise training for patients with amyotrophic lateral sclerosis: A systematic review and meta-analysis. Physiotherapy. 2021;**113**:12-28

www.ingramcontent.com/pod-product-compliance
Lightning Source LLC
Chambersburg PA
CBHW081228190326
41458CB00016B/5717